Introduction to Statistics for Forensic Scientists

Introduction to Statistics for Forensic Scientists

David Lucy
University of Edinburgh, UK

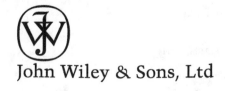

John Wiley & Sons, Ltd

Other Wiley Editorial Offices

John Wiley & Sons Inc., 111 River Street, Hoboken, NJ 07030, USA

Jossey-Bass, 989 Market Street, San Francisco, CA 94103-1741, USA

Wiley-VCH Verlag GmbH, Boschstr. 12, D-69469 Weinheim, Germany

John Wiley & Sons Australia Ltd, 33 Park Road, Milton, Queensland 4064, Australia

John Wiley & Sons (Asia) Pte Ltd, 2 Clementi Loop #02-01, Jin Xing Distripark, Singapore 129809

John Wiley & Sons Canada Ltd, 22 Worcester Road, Etobicoke, Ontario, Canada M9W 1L1

Wiley also publishes its books in a variety of electronic formats. Some content that appears in print may not
be available in electronic books.

Library of Congress Cataloging-in-Publication Data

Lucy, David.
   Introduction to statistics for forensic scientists / David Lucy.
     p. cm.
   Includes bibliographical references and index.
   ISBN 0-470-02200-0—ISBN 0-470-02201-9
1. Forensic sciences–Statistical methods.   2. Forensic statistics.   3. Evidence (Law)–Statistical methods.
I. Title.
   HV8073.L83 2005
   519.5024′36325   2005028184

British Library Cataloguing in Publication Data

A catalogue record for this book is available from the British Library

ISBN-13 978-0-470-2200-0 (HB) ISBN-13 978-0-470-02201 9 (PB)
ISBN-10 0-470-2200-0 (HB)   ISBN-10 0-470-02201 9 (PB)

Typeset in 10.5/13pt Times and Officina by TechBooks, New Delhi, India

Contents

Preface

The detective story, whether it be in the form of a novel, a television programme, or a cinema film, has always exerted a fascination for people from all walks of life. Much of the appeal of the detective story lies in the way in which a series of seemingly disconnected observations fit a narrative structure where all pieces of information are eventually revealed to the reader, or viewer, make a whole and logical nexus. The story which emerges by the end of the plot as to how, and just as importantly why, the perpetrator committed the crime, is shown by some device, such as a confession by the "guilty" character, to be a true description of the circumstances surrounding the crime.

Detective stories have, at their core, some important and fundamental truths about how humans perceive what is true from what is false. The logical arguments used are woven together with elements of evidence taken from widely differing types of observation. Some observations will be hearsay, others may be more material observations such as blood staining. All these facts will be put together in some logical way to create a case against one of the characters in the story.

However, detective stories do have a tendency to neglect one of the more important elements of real investigation. That element is uncertainty. The interpretation of real observations is usually subject to uncertainty, for example, the bloodstain on the carpet may "match" the suspect in some biochemical way, but was the blood which made the bloodstain derived from the suspect, or one of the other possible individuals who could be described as a "match". Statistical science is the science of uncertainty, and it is only appropriate that statistics should provide at least part of the answer to some of the uncertain parts of evidence encountered in criminal investigations. That part of evidence upon which it is possible to throw some illumination is that evidence generated by forensic scientists. This tends to be numerical by nature, and is thus amenable to analysis by statisticians.

The are though, two roles for statistics in forensic science. The first is a need for forensic scientists to be able to take their laboratory data from experiments, and interpret that data in the same way that any observational scientist would do. This strand of statistical knowledge is commonly used by all sorts of scientists, and guides to it can be found in any handbook of applied statistical methods. The second role of statistical science is in the interpretation of observations from the case work with which forensic scientist may become involved. This strand of application of statistical methods in forensic science has been termed evidence evaluation. These days a number of books exist outlining statistical evidence evaluation techniques, all of them excellent, but unfortunately none of them aimed towards those who are relatively new to statistical science, and require a certain technical insight into the subject.

This volume attempts to bridge the gap in the literature by commencing with the use of statistics to analyse data generated during laboratory experiments, then progressing to address the issue of how observations made by, and reported to the forensic scientist may be considered as evidence.

Finally, I should like to acknowledge the assistance of Bruce Worton, Colin Aitken, Breedette Hayes, Gzregorz Zadora, James Curran, Nicola Martin, Nicola Clayson, Mandy Jay, Franco Taroni, John Kingston, Dave Barclay, Tom Nelson and Burkhard Schaffer. R (R development core team, 2004) was used to create all diagrams and calculations which appear in this volume. My gratitude is also due to all those forensic scientists who have allowed me the use of their data in this volume.

List of figures

List of tables

1 A short history of statistics in the law

The science of statistics refers to two distinct, but linked, areas of knowledge. The first is the enumeration of types of event and counts of entities for economic, social and scientific purposes, the second is the examination of uncertainty. It is in this second guise that statistics can be regarded as the science of uncertainty. It is therefore natural that statistics should be applied to evidence used for legal purposes as uncertainty is a feature of any legal process where decisions are made upon the basis of evidence. Typically, if a case is brought to a court it is the role of the court to discern, using evidence, what has happened, then decide what, if anything, has to be done in respect of the alleged events. Courts in the common law tradition are not in themselves bodies which can directly launch investigations into events, but are institutions into which evidence is brought for decisions to be made. Unless all the evidence points unambiguously towards an inevitable conclusion, different pieces of evidence will carry different implications with varying degrees of force. Modern statistical methods are available which are designed to measure this 'weight' of evidence.

1.1 History

Informal notions of probability have been a feature of decision making which date to at least as far in the past as the earliest writing. Many applications were, as related by Franklin (2001), to the process of law. Ancient Egypt seems to have two strands, one of which relates to the number of reliable witnesses willing to testify for or against a case, evidence which remains important today. The other is the use of oracles and is no longer in use. Even in the ancient world there seems to have been scepticism about the information divulged by oracles, sometimes two or three being consulted and the majority opinion followed. Subsequently the Jewish tradition made the assessment of uncertainty central to many religious and legal

Introduction to Statistics for Forensic Scientists   David Lucy
© 2005 John Wiley & Sons, Ltd.

practices. Jewish law is notable in that it does not admit confession, a wholly worthy feature which makes torture useless. It also required a very high standard of proof which differed according to the seriousness of any alleged offence. Roman law had the concept of onus of proof, but the wealthier sections of Roman society were considered more competent to testify then others. The Roman judiciary were allowed some latitude to judge in accordance with the evidence. In contrast to Jewish law, torture was widespread in Roman practice. In fact in some circles the evidence from a tortured witness was considered of a higher quality than had the same witness volunteered the evidence, particularly if they happened to be a member of the slave classes.

European Medieval law looked to the Roman codes, but started to take a more abstract view of law based on general principles. This included developments in the theory of evidence such as half, quarter and finer grades of proof, and multiple supporting strands forming what we today would call a case. There seem to have been variable attitudes to the use of torture. Ordeal was used in the earlier period to support the civil law in cases which were otherwise intractable. An important tool for evidence evaluation with its beginnings in the Western European Medieval was the development of a form of jury which has continued uninterrupted until the present day. It is obvious that the ancient thinkers had some idea that the evidence with which they were dealing was uncertain, and devised many ingenious methods of making some sort of *best* decision in the face of the uncertainties, usually revolving around some weighting scheme given to the various individual pieces of evidence, and some process of summation. Nevertheless, it is apparent that uncertainty was not thought about in the same way in which we would think about it today.

Informal enumeration types of analyses were applied as early as in the middle of the 17th century to observational data with John Gaunt's analysis of the London Mortality bills (Gaunt, 1662, cited in Stigler, 1986), and it is at this point in time that French mathematicians such as De Méré, Roberval, Pascal and Fermet started to work on a more recognizably modern notion of probability in their attempts to solve the problem of how best to divide up the stakes on interrupted dice games.

From there, ideas of mathematical probability were steadily developed into all areas of science using large run, or frequentist, type approaches. They were also applied to law, finding particular uses in civil litigation in the United States of America where the methods of statistics have been used, and continue to be used, to aid courts in their deliberations in such areas as employment discrimination and antitrust legislation (Fienberg, 1988).

First suggested in the latter part of the nineteenth century by Poincaré, Darboux and Appell (Aitken and Taroni, 2004, p. 153) was an intuitive and intellectually satisfying method for placing a simple value on evidence. This employed a measure called a likelihood ratio, and was the beginning of a more modern approach to evidence evaluation in forensic science. A likelihood ratio is a statistical method which can be used directly to assess the worth of observations, and is currently the predominant measure for numerically based evidence.

Since the inception of DNA evidence in forensic science in the courts of the mid 1980s, lawyers, and indeed forensic scientists themselves, have looked towards statistical science to provide precise evaluation of the worth of evidence which follows the explicitly probabilistic approach to the evidential value of DNA matches.

1.2 Some recent uses of statistics in forensic science

A brief sample of the *Journal of Forensic Sciences* between the years 1999 and 2002 shows that about half of the papers have some sort of statistical content. These can be classified into: regression and calibration, percentages, classical hypothesis tests, means, standard deviations, classification and other methods. This makes knowledge of numerical techniques at some level essential, either for publication in the literature, or knowledgeable and informed reading.

The statistical methods used in the surveyed papers were:

1. Regression and calibration – regression is finding the relationship between one thing and another. For example, Thompson *et al.* (1999) wished to compare amounts of explosive residue detected by GC-MS with that detected by LC-UV. To do this they undertook a regression analysis which told them that the relationship was almost 1:1, that is, they would have more or less the same measurement from either method. Calibration is in some senses the complement of regression in that what you are trying to do is make an estimate of one quantity from another. Migeot and De Kinder (2002) used calibration to make estimates of how many shots an assault rifle had fired since its piston was last cleaned by the number of carbon particles on the piston.

2. Percentages and enumeration statistics – counts and proportions of objects, employed universally as summary statistics.

3. Means, standard deviations and *t*-tests – a mean is a measure of location[†]. For example, Solari and Abramovitch (2002) used stages in the development of teeth to estimate ages for Hispanic detainees in Texas. They assigned known age individuals to 10 stages of third molar development and calculated the mean age for the individuals falling in that age category. What they were then able to do was to assign any unknown individual to a developmental category, thus suggesting an expected age for that individual.

   Standard deviations are measures of dispersion about a mean. In the example above, Solari and Abramovitch (2002) also calculated the standard deviation for age for each of their developmental categories. They were then able to gain some idea of how wrong they would be in assigning any age to an unknown individual.

[†] Location in this context is a measure of any central tendency, for instance, male stature in the United Kingdom tends towards 5′8″.

t-tests tell you how different are two samples based on the means and standard deviations of those samples. For example, Koons and Buscaglia (2002) used *t*-tests on elemental compositions from glass found at a crime scene to that found on a suspect to tell whether the two samples of glass possibly came from the same source.

4. Classification – this allows the researcher to assign categories on the basis of some measurement. Stojanowski and Siedemann (1999) used neck bone measurements from known sex skeletons and a discriminant function analysis to calculate a feature rule which would allow them to categorize skeletal remains as male, or female.

5. Other methods – these include χ^2[‡] tests and Bayesian methods.

1.3 What is probability?

When we speak of probability what is it we mean? Everybody uses the expression 'probably' to express belief favouring one possible outcome, or world state, over other possible outcomes, but does the term probability confer other meanings?

Examining the sorts of things which constitute mathematical ideas of probability there seem to be two different sorts. The first are the aleatory[§] probabilities, such events as the outcomes from dice throwing and coin tossing. Here the system is known, and the probabilities deduced from knowledge of the system. For instance, with a fair coin I know that in any single toss it will land with probability 0.5 heads, and probability 0.5 tails. I also know that in a long run of tosses roughly half will be heads, and roughly half tails.

A second type of probability is epistemic. This is where we have no innate knowledge of the system from which to deduce probabilities for outcomes, but can by observation induce knowledge of the system. Suppose one were to examine a representative number of people and found that 60% of them were mobile telephone users. Then we would have some knowledge of the structure of mobile telephone ownership amongst the population, but because we had not examined every member of the population to see whether or not they were a mobile telephone user, our estimate based on those we had looked at would be subject to a quantifiable uncertainty.

Scientists often use this sort type of generalization to suggest possible mechanisms which underly the observations. This type of empiricism employs, by necessity, some form of the uniformitarian assumption. The uniformitarian assumption implies that processes observed in the present will have been in operation in the past, and will be in operation in the future. A form of the uniformitarian assumption is, to some extent, an inevitable feature of all sciences based upon observation, but it is the absolute

---

[‡] Pronounced 'chi-squared'.
[§] Aleatory just means by chance and is not a word specific to statistics.

cornerstone of statistics. Without accepting the assumption that the processes which cause some members of a population to take on certain characteristics are at work in the wider population, any form of statistical inference, or estimation, is impossible.

To what extent probabilities from induced and deduced systems are different is open to some debate. The deduced probability cannot ever be applied to anything other than a notional system. A die may be specified as fair, but any real die will always have minor inconsistencies and flaws which will make it not quite fair. To some extent the aleatory position is artificial and tautological. When a fair die is stipulated then we know the properties in some absolute sense of the die. It is not possible to have this absolute knowledge about any actual observable system. We simply use the notion as a convenient framework from which to develop a calculus of probability, which, whenever it is used, must be applied to probability systems which are fundamentally epistemic. Likewise, because all inferences made about populations are based on the observation of a few members of that population, some degree of deduced aleatory uncertainty is inevitable as part of that inference.

As all real probabilities are induced by observation, and are essentially frequencies, does this mean that a probability can only ever be a statement about the relative proportions of observations in a population? And, if so, is it nonsense to speak of the probability for a single event of special interest?

An idea of a frequency being attached to an outcome for a single event is ridiculous as the outcome of interest either happens or does not happen, From a single throw of a six-sided die we cannot have an outcome in which the die lands 1/6 with its six face uppermost, it either lands with the six face uppermost, or it does not. There is no possible physical state of affairs which correspond to a probability of 1/6 for a single event. Were one to throw the six-sided die 12 times then the physical state corresponding to a probability of 1/6 would be the observation of two sixes. But there can be no single physical event which corresponds to a probability of 1/6.

The only way in which a single event can be quantified by a probability is to conceive of that probability as a product of mind, in short to hold an idealist interpretation of probability (Hacking, 1966). This is what statisticians call subjective probability (O'Hagen, 2004) and is an interpretation of probability which stipulates that probability is a function of, and only exists in, the mind of those interested in the event in question. This is why they are subjective, not because they are somehow unfounded or made up, but because they rely upon idealist interpretations of probability.

A realist interpretation of probability would be one which is concerned with frequencies and numbers of outcomes in long runs of events, and making inferences about the proportions of outcomes in wider populations. A realist interpretation of probability would not be able to make statements about the outcome of a single event as any such statement must necessarily be a belief as it cannot exist in the observable world, and therefore requires some ideal notion of probability. Realist positions imply that there is something in the observed world which is causing uncertainty, uncertainty being a property external to the mind of the observer. Some might argue that these external probabilities are propensities of the system in question to behave in a specific way. Unfortunately the propensity theory of probability generates the same problem for a realist conception when applied to a single event because a propensity cannot be observed directly, and would have to be a product of mind. In many respects realist interpretations can be more productive for the scientist because of the demands that some underlying explanatory factor be hypothesized or found. This is in contrast to idealist positions where a cause for uncertainty is desirable, but not absolutely necessary, as the uncertainty resides in the mind.

This distinction between realist and idealist is not one which is seen in statistical sciences, and indeed the terms are not used. There are no purely realist statisticians; all statisticians are willing to make probabilistic statements about single events, so all statisticians are to some degree idealistic about their conception of probability. However, a debate in statistics which mirrors the realist/idealist positions is that of the frequentist/Bayesian approaches. There is a mathematical theorem of probability called Bayes' theorem, which we will encounter in Section 9.2, and Bayesians are a school of statisticians named after the theorem. The differences between Bayesians and frequentists are not mathematical, Bayes' theorem is a mathematical theorem and, given the tenets of probability theory, Bayes' theorem is correct. The differences are in this interpretation of the nature of probability. Frequentists tend to argue against subjective probabilities, and for long-run frequency based interpretations of probability. Bayesians are in favour of subjective notions of probability, and think that all quantities which are uncertain can be expressed in probabilistic terms.

This leads to a rather interesting position for forensic scientists. On the one hand they do experimental work in the laboratory where long runs of repeated results are possible; on the other hand they have to interpret data as evidence which relates to singular events. The latter aspect of the work of the forensic scientist is explicitly idealistic because events in a criminal or civil case happened once and only once, and require a subjective interpretation of probability to interpret probabilities as degrees of belief. The experimental facet of forensic science can easily accommodate a more realist view of probability.

The subjective view of probability is the one which most easily fits common-sense notions of probability, and the only one which can be used to quantify uncertainty about single events. There are some fears amongst scientists that a subjective probability is an undemonstrated probability without foundation or empirical support, and indeed a subjective probability can be that. But most subjective probabilities are based on frequencies observed empirically, and are not, as the term subjective might imply, somehow snatched out of the air, or made up.

There is a view of the nature of probability which can side-step many of the problems and debates about the deeper meaning of just what probability is. This is an instrumentalist position (Hacking, 1966) where one simply does not care about the exact interpretation of probability, but rather one simply views it as a convenient intellectual devise to enable calculations to be made about uncertainty. The instrumentalist's position implies a loosely idealist background, where probability is a product of mind, and not a fundamental component of the material world.

2 Data types, location and dispersion

All numeric data can be classified into one or more types. For most types of data the most basic descriptive statistics are a measure of central tendency, called location, and some measure of dispersion, which to some extent is a measure of how good is a description the measure of central tendency. The concepts of location and dispersion do not apply to all data types.

2.1 Types of data

There are three fundamental types of data:

1. *Nominal* data are simply classified into discrete categories, the ordering having no significance. Biological sex usually comes in male/female, whereas gender can be male/female/other. Things such as drugs can be classified by geographical area such as South American, Afghan, Northern Indian or Oriental. Further descriptions by some measure of location, and dispersion, are not really relevant to data of this type.

2. *Ordinal* data are again classified into discrete categories; this time the ordering does have significance. The development of the third molar (Solari and Abramovitch, 2002) was classified into 10 stages. Each class related to age, and therefore the order in which the classes appear is important.

3. *Continuous* data types can take on any value in an allowed range. The concentration of magnesium in glass is a continuous data type which can range from 0% to about 5% before the glass becomes a substance which is not glass. Within that range magnesium can adopt any value such as 1.225% or 0.856%.

Introduction to Statistics for Forensic Scientists   David Lucy
© 2005 John Wiley & Sons, Ltd.

Table 2.1 Table of year and Δ^9-THC (%) for marijuana seizures: these data are simulated (with permission) from ElSohly *et al.* (2001) and are more fully listed in Table 2.2

Seizure	Year	Δ^9-THC (%)
1	1986	9.26
2	1987	7.58
3	1987	7.65
4	1986	10.29
5	1986	8.29
6	1987	7.85
7	1986	8.40
⋮	⋮	⋮

Table 2.2 Table of year and Δ^9-THC (%) for marijuana seizures: these data are simulated (with permission) from ElSohly *et al.* (2001)

Year	Δ^9-THC (%)	
1986	9.26	10.30
	8.29	8.40
	8.32	8.84
	8.82	8.41
	9.74	9.02
	10.70	7.05
	7.91	7.72
	8.41	8.93
	7.21	9.95
	6.29	8.16
1987	7.59	7.66
	7.85	7.91
	6.61	7.42
	6.91	8.46
	8.34	8.12
	7.97	7.15
	9.09	7.93
	7.93	

The type of data sometimes restricts the approaches which can be used to examine and make inferences about those data. For example, the idea of central tendency, and a dispersion about the central tendency, is not really relevant to nominal data, whereas both can be used to summarize ordinal and continuous data types.

There are a few of points of terminology with which it is necessary to be familiar:

- Nominal and ordinal data types are known collectively as *discrete*, because they place entities into discrete exclusive categories.

- All the above data types are called *variables*.

- There are nominal and ordinal (occasionally continuous) variables which are used to classify other variables, these are called *factors*. An example would be Δ^9-THC concentrations in marijuana seizures from various years in the 1980s given in Table 2.1. Here '% Δ^9-THC' is a continuous *variable* and 'year' is an *ordinal variable* which is being used as a *factor* to classify Δ^9-THC.

2.2 Populations and samples

Generally in chemistry, biology and other natural sciences a sample is something taken for the purposes of examination, for example a fibre and a piece of glass may be found at the scene of a crime; these would be termed samples. In statistics a sample has a different meaning. It is a sub-set of a larger set, known as a population. In the table of dates and % Δ^9-THC in Table 2.1, the % Δ^9-THC column gives measurements of the % Δ^9-THC in a sample of marijuana seizures at the corresponding date. In this case the population is marijuana seizures.

Populations and samples must be hierarchically arranged. For instance one could examine the 1986 entries and this would be a sample of % Δ^9-THC in a 1986 population of marijuana seizures. It could also be said that the sample was a sample of the population of all marijuana seizures, albeit a small one. Were all marijuana observed for 1986 this would be the population of marijuana for 1986, which could for some purposes be regarded as a sample of all marijuana from the population of marijuana from the 1980s. The population of marijuana from the 1980s could be seen as a sample of marijuana from the 20th century.

It is important to realize that the notions of population and sample are not fixed in nature, but are defined by the entities under examination, and the purposes to which observation of those entities is to be put. However, populations and samples are always hierarchically arranged in that a sample is always a sub-set of a population.

2.3 Distributions

Most generally a distribution is an arrangement of frequencies of some observation in a meaningful order. If all 20 values for THC content of 1986 marijuana seizures are grouped into broad categories, that is the continuous variable % THC is made into an ordinal variable with many values, then the frequencies of THC content in each category can be tabulated. This table can be represented graphically as a histogram[†].

A histogram of simulated Δ^9-THC frequencies from 1986 taken from Table 2.2, is represented in Figure 2.1. In Figure 2.1 the horizontal axis is divided into 14 categories of 0.5% each, the vertical axis is labelled 0 to 10, and indicates the counts, or frequency, of occurrences in that particular category. So for the first two categories (5 → 6%) there are no values, the second category (6.0 → 6.5%) occurs with a frequency 1, and so on.

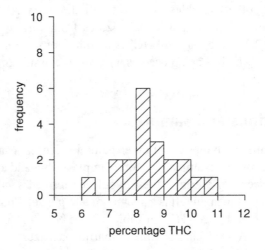

Figure 2.1 Histogram of simulated Δ^9-THC (%) values for a sample of marijuana seizures dating from 1986

The histogram in Figure 2.1, which gives the sample frequency *distribution* for Δ^9-THC in marijuana from 1986, has three important properties:

1. It has a single highest point at about 8.25% THC, the two ends of the distribution (tails) having progressively lower frequencies as they get further from the highest point. This property is called *unimodal* and indicates that there is some tendency amongst 1986 marijuana consignments towards a THC content of about 8.25%.

2. The distribution is more or less symmetric about the 8.25% value.

3. The distribution is dispersed about the 8.25% point in some measurable way.

The histogram in Figure 2.2 is the sample distribution for THC in marijuana from 1987. Here the % THC tends towards a value of about 7.75%; the same properties of dispersion about this value and a sort of symmetry can be seen as in Figure 2.1.

[†] A histogram is not to be confused with a bar chart, which looks similar, but in a bar chart height represents frequency rather than the area of the rectangles. Usually in a histogram the categories are of equal 'width', but this is not always the case.

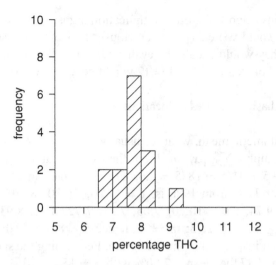

Figure 2.2 Histogram of simulated Δ^9-THC (%) values for a sample of marijuana seizures dating from 1987

Both the above distributions are termed unimodal because they are symmetric about a single maximal value. If two distinct peaks were visible then the distribution would be termed bimodal, more than two multimodal.

We have seen above from Figures 2.1 and 2.2 that the percentage Δ^9-THC from marijuana seized in 1986 will typically be about 8.25% (Figure 2.1) and that from 1987 about 7.25%. How do we then go about measuring the 'typical' quantities, and the dispersions?

2.4 Location

First some mathematical notation and terminology is required:

- Let x be an *array* such that $x = \{2, 4, 3, 5, 4\}$. This means that x is a series of quantities called an array which are indexed by the suffix i, so that $x_1 = 2$, $x_2 = 4$, $x_3 = 3$ and so on.

- n is the number of elements in array x. In this case there are five elements in x so that $x_n = x_5 = 4$. n is a single number on its own and is sometimes referred to as a *scalar*.

- $\sum_{i=1}^{n} x_i$ is the summation of all the elements from x_1 to x_n ($\sum$ is S in Greek and indicates summation). For x this would be: $\sum_{i=1}^{n} x_i = x_1 + x_2 + \ldots + x_5 = 2 + 4 + 3 + 5 + 4 = 18$. $\sum_{i=1}^{3} x_i$ would be $x_1 + x_2 + x_3 = 2 + 4 + 3 = 9$. A more complicated example is: $\sum_{i=1}^{3}(x_i + 1)$ which evaluates as $(x_1 + 1) + (x_2 + 1) + (x_3 + 1) = (2 + 1) + (4 + 1) + (3 + 1) = 3 + 5 + 4 = 12$.

- Mathematicians often leave out multiplication signs, so rather than writing $3 \times x_1 = 6$, they would write $3x_1 = 6$. Obviously if two numerical constants are in conjunction they would usually be evaluated, but if they are not a $\times$ sign would be employed. For example $3 \times 4 = 12$ would never be written $34 = 12$.

There are three basic measures of location:

1. *Mean* the arithmetic mean, what we usually think of as an average. Denoted as $\bar{x}$ which is simply $(\sum_{i=1}^{n} x_i)/n$. From the example above, $\bar{x} = (\sum_{i=1}^{n} x_i)/n = (2 + 4 + 3 + 5 + 4)/5 = 18/5 = 3.6$. For example, in the 1986 marijuana example x for THC from 1986 is: $x = \{9.26,\ 10.30,\ 8.29,\ 8.40,\ 8.32,\ 8.84,\ 8.82,\ 8.41,\ 9.74,\ 9.02,\ 10.70,\ 7.05,\ 7.91,\ 7.72,\ 8.41,\ 8.93,\ 7.21, 9.95, 6.29, 8.16\}$, so $\sum_{i=1}^{n} x_i = 171.73$; $n = 20$, hence $\bar{x} = 8.59\%$ rather than the 8.25% estimated from inspection of the histogram. Performing the same calculation for the data from 1987 the mean is 7.80% with $n = 15$.

2. *Median* is simply the value of the middle one of a number of vectors ordered in increasing magnitude. In the example (above) $x = \{2, 4, 3, 5, 4\}$, let x' be an ordered vector of x so that $x' = \{2, 3, 4, 4, 5\}$, as n is $5^{\ddagger}$ then the centre value is 3, so the median is $x'_3 = 4$. The medians for THC from 1986 and 1987 are 8.41 and 7.91 respectively which are quite close to the means and indicate symmetry.

3. *Mode* is the value with most instances. In $x = \{2, 4, 3, 5, 4\}$ there are two occurrences of 4, so 4 is the modal value. Technically for the THC concentration data all values are on a continuous scale, so there are no repeats. However, if these data are grouped, as with the histograms, then from Figure 2.1 the modal group for the sample from 1986 is the one with the tallest column. This corresponds to a value of 8.25, that from 1987 (from Figure 2.2) being 7.75, and is equivalent to that estimated by inspection.

Using the correct measure of location is important, usually this will be the mean, but sometimes the median and mode are also the most appropriate measures of location. For instance, the use of the mean rather than the median as a measure of income may indicate salaries are higher than they actually are for most people. Let $x = \{£12,000, £20,000, £21,000, £11,000, £9,000, £7,000, £13,000, £85,000, £120,000\}$ be an array representing salaries in units of £ then $\bar{x} = £33,111$, however, the median is only £13,000. However, it is quite legitimate to describe the average income as £33,111, only two out of nine earn any more than this, and in fact one would expect most people to be earning less than £13,000, as five of the nine earn less than £13,000. So a more appropriate measure of location might be the median value. The distribution seen in Figure 2.3 is known as a skewed distribution, in this case highly skewed towards the higher values of income (positively skewed).

$\ddagger$ For even n split the difference of the two middle values. That is, if $n = 4$ take the mean of x_2 and x_3.

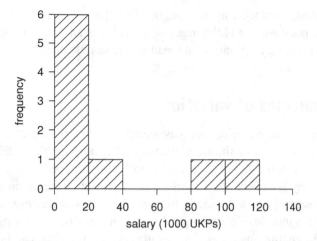

Figure 2.3 A histogram of salaries which is heavily skewed towards the lower range

2.5 Dispersion

In Section 2.3 we looked at some distributions by use of the histogram, and in Section 2.4 measures of typical values, or location, for those distributions were calculated. This section focuses on a measure of dispersion of a given distribution about a typical measure.

The standard measure of dispersion is called *variance*[§]. Consider $x = \{2, 4, 3, 5, 4\}$, then $\bar{x} = 3.6$. The distance between x_1 and $\bar{x}$ is $x_1 - \bar{x} = 2 - 3.6 = -1.6$.

Let x' be a vector of distances between x and $\bar{x}$. Repeating the above process of examining the distances between x_i and $\bar{x}$, for $x_{2 \to n}$, we get $x' = \{-1.6, 0.4, -0.6, 1.4, 0.4\}$.

Summing these gives an answer of 0 because all the negative values cancel all the positive values, so this would not be a useful measure of dispersion. However, if we square all the distances between the mean of x and the values of x, we obtain a measure which when summed will not be zero because all the negative values become positive values by the process of squaring.

Squaring and summing for x' we have $(x')^2 = \{2.56, 0.16, 0.36, 1.96, 0.16\}$ and $\sum_{i=1}^{n}(x')^2 = 5.20$.

Obviously the greater n the value of, the larger $\sum_{i=1}^{n}(x')^2$ will become regardless of the dispersion properties of x. To correct for the size of n, the sum of the squared differences is simply divided by $n - 1$ to obtain the variance of x; i.e. variance of $x = 5.2/(5 - 1) = 5.2/4 = 1.3$. In mathematical notation:

$$\text{variance}\,(x) = \frac{\sum_{i=1}^{n}(x_i - \bar{x})^2}{n - 1}$$

[§] There are others such as inter-quartile ranges, but they will not be covered here.

At its simplest, variance can be thought of as the average of squared deviations between the points of x and the mean of x, which is an scaled by $n - 1$ to correct the bias of replacing the population mean by the sample mean.

2.6 Hierarchies of variation

Measurements from empirical sources are nearly always subject to some level of variability. This can be as simple as the variability attributable to different years as we have seen with the Δ^9-THC levels in marijuana seizures data. The lowest level in the hierarchy is observational variability, that is an observation is made on the same entity several times in exactly the same way, and those observations are seen to vary. The magnitude of observational variability may be zero for discrete variable types, but for continuous types, such as glass measurements, can be considerable. The next level up is within entity variability, where the same entity is repeatedly measured, but varying the way in which it is measured. For something such as glass compositional measurements different fragments from the same pane of glass might be measured. Within sample variability is where different entities from the same sample are observed and found to vary. This too may be zero for discrete variable types. It goes without saying that these can be between sample variability.

These stages in this hierarchy of variation tend to be additive. For instance, if the THC content is measured for the 1986 sample, then because the measurement are made on different consignments in the same sample, the variance of all the measurements will represent the sum of the first three levels of variability. The variance from both the 1986 and 1987 samples, when taken together, will be the sum of all the levels of variance in the hierarchy. Some statistical methods use estimates of variance from different sources to make statements about the data, but these are beyond the scope of this book.

Review questions

1. What sort of variable is a DNA profile?

2. I have made five measurements of refractive index from each of 20 fragments of glass from a single window pane. What are the samples and populations of this hierarchical structure.

3. Is the distribution of heights of women in the UK unimodal?

4. Is the distribution of heights of adults in the UK unimodal?

5. As what variable type is sex being as in the above two questions?

6. Let $x = \{16, 17, 21, 21, 21, 23, 23\}$

    (a) Evaluate $x_1 + x_3$.
    (b) Evaluate $\sum_1^3 x$.
    (c) Evaluate $\bar{x}$.
    (d) What is the median of x.
    (e) What is the mode of x.
    (f) What is the variance of x.

3 Probability

Even though there is no complete agreement about the fundamental nature of probability amongst statisticians and probability theorists, there is a body of elementary probability theory about which all agree. The fundamental principle is that the probability for any event is between 0 and 1 inclusive, that is, for any event A $0 \leq \Pr(A) \leq 1$ where Pr stands for probability, and the element in the parentheses is the event under consideration. This is the *first law of probability*, sometimes known as the *convexity rule*, and implies occurs with probability of event which cannot happen, an event which occurs with probability 1 is an event which must happen, and events which occur with probabilities between 0 and 1 are subject to some degree of uncertainty.

3.1 Aleatory probability

Aleatory[†] probabilities are the calculation of probabilities where those probabilities can be notionally deduced from the physical nature of the system generating the uncertainty in outcome with which we are concerned. Such systems include fair coins, fair dice and random drawing from packs of cards. Many of the basic ideas of probability theory are derived from, and can best be described by these simple randomization devices.

One throw of a six-sided die

If I have a fair die the probability of throwing a six from a single throw is 1 in 6 or $1/6 = 0.17$ or 17%. There are six faces on a fair dice, numbered $1, \ldots, 6$, any of which in a single throw is equally likely to end face up, and is certain that the die

[†] Aleatory just means by chance and is not a word specific to statistics.

Introduction to Statistics for Forensic Scientists   David Lucy
© 2005 John Wiley & Sons, Ltd.

must end its roll with one face uppermost. The event in which we are interested is the outcome of a six facing uppermost. Stating this intuition as an equation:

$$Pr(E) = \frac{\text{number of ways in which E can occur}}{\text{number of ways in which all equally likely events can occur including E}}$$

For the dice there is one way in which a six can be thrown, and six ways in which a dice can land, therefore $Pr(A) = 1/6$, or 17%.

If the event of interest is the probability of *not* throwing a six then we know there are five ways in which a fair six-sided die can be thrown, and a six not land uppermost. There are six equally likely ways in which a fair die can land, and exactly one face must land uppermost. Therefore $Pr(B) = 5/6 = 0.83$, where B is the probability of throwing 1 or 2 or 3 or 4 or 5.

There is another way of calculating this probability. The probability of throwing a six is $1/6$, the probability of throwing any number is 1, so the probability of throwing anything but a six is $1 - 1/6 = 5/6 = 0.83$. This event of throwing anything but a six can be denoted as $\overline{A}$ where the line over the A denotes *not*, a, thus $\overline{A}$ and B are the same event which occur with the same probability.

The probability $Pr(A)$ of throwing a six on a fair die is $Pr(A) = 1/6$. $Pr(\overline{A})$ is the probability of throwing anything but a six, where the event E is again the event of throwing a six. As a single die must land with exactly one face uppermost, a single throw must result in a six, or not a six, so:

$$Pr(E) + Pr(\overline{E}) = 1$$

which is known as the *first law of probability*, and is simply another way of saying that at least one of the possible events must happen.

A single throw with more than one outcome of interest

If we wish to calculate the probability of throwing a two *or* six we can go about it in more or less the same way. There is one way in which a two can be thrown from a single die, and one way in which a six can be thrown, so if C is the event of a two *or* six being thrown, then there are two ways in which this can happen, and six equally likely possible outcomes, so $Pr(C) = 2/6 = 1/3 = 0.33$.

This can be considered the combination of the two individual probabilities. Statisticians and probability theorists are always interested in reducing the calculation of more complex probabilities to multiple calculations of simpler probabilities. If A is the event of throwing a six, and B the event of throwing a two, then we know $Pr(A) = 1/6$, and $Pr(B) = 1/6$, so if E is throwing a 2, or 6, then $Pr(E) = Pr(A) + Pr(B) = 1/6 + 1/6 = 2/6 = 1/3 = 0.33$.

The same calculation can be applied to the complement of this. Consider $\overline{D}$ as the event of throwing a 1, 3, 4, 5 then $Pr(\overline{D}) = 1/6 + 1/6 + 1/6 + 1/6 = 4/6$, or as $1 - Pr(D) = 1 - 2/6 = 4/6$.

More generally:

$$\Pr(A \text{ or } B) = \Pr(A) + \Pr(B) \tag{1}$$

This is known as the *second law of probability*, and this version only holds for what are known as mutually exclusive events. From a single die throw the events of throwing a five and six are mutually exclusive as it is not possible to throw a five and a six from a single throw, but only a five or a six. The possible events from a single die throw are also termed exhaustive. That is, it is only possible to throw a 1, 2, 3, 4, 5, or 6. It is not possible to throw any other score, and by enumerating 1 through to 6 we have exhaustively described the possible events from a single throw of a six-sided die.

Two six-sided dice

If two fair dice, or two throws of the same fair die are considered, what is the probability of throwing a 5, then a 6?

Let A denote the throwing of a 5 from the first die. There is only one way in which a five can be followed by a six in two throws of a die, and that for each of the six outcomes of the first die, there are a possible six outcomes from the second die, making a total of 36 possible distinct outcomes, thus $\Pr(E) = 1/36 \approx 0.03 \approx 3\%$ where E is the joint event of a five followed by a six. A joint event is the term used for an event made of two simpler events occuring simultaneously. In the case described here the simple events are the throwing of a five, and the throwing of a six. The joint event is the combined event of throwing of a five, then a six.

We can also consider this as the product of the single event probabilities. If $\Pr(A) = 1/6$ where A is the probability of throwing a five with the first die, and $\Pr(B) = 1/6$ with the second then:

$$\Pr(A, B) = \Pr(A) \times \Pr(B)$$

where $\Pr(A, B)$ means the probability of joint event A *and* B. This is sometimes called the *product rule*, or *the third law of probability* and is used to calculate probabilities for joint events which are *independent*. Independence in this case means that one event has no influence whatsoever on the other event in anyway at all. Here the first throw of the dice cannot influence the outcome of the second, or *vice versa*, therefore they are independent events. For most events in systems which are not described by simple systems such as card games, or dice throwing, independence cannot be presumed, and often is not the case. For instance, were there a probability of $1/10$ for the event of encountering a male with a beard, and a $1/10$ probability of encountering a male with a moustache there would *not* be a $1/100$ probability of encountering a male with a moustache and beard, because nearly all males with beards also have moustaches, and many males with moustaches also have beards. The events of 'male with moustache' and 'male with beard' are not independent and we cannot use the product rule to work out probabilities for the joint event. Instead we must reformulate the *third law of probability* to account for the dependence between events.

Dependent events

Even with a simple aleatory system such as the throwing of a die not all events can be considered to be independent. Consider two events, A is the throwing of an odd number from a fair six-sided die which, as there are three odd numbers, will occur $Pr(A) = 1/2$. Let B be the throwing of a number greater than three from the same die, there are three numbers greater than three on a six-sided die, so that $P(B) = 1/2$. These two events are not independent in that it is possible to throw a number greater than three which is odd, namely the throwing of a five which is the probability of A and B or $Pr(A$ and $B) = 1/6$. If we were to consider the two events as independent then we might incorrectly calculate a probability of $1/4$ by multiplying $1/2 \times 1/2$ for the joint event of an odd number greater than 3.

In the example above, the outcomes for A are $\{1, 3, 5\}$ which are all the odd numbers available from a six-sided die. Let us imagine that A has already happened and we have rolled an odd number, and this has occurred with probability $1/2$. Given this fact, what is the probability that the odd number we have rolled is greater than 3? There are three outcomes for A, that is $\{1, 3, 5\}$, only one of which, five, is greater than three, so *given* we have rolled an odd number the probability that it is greater than three is $1/3$.

So we have calculated the probability of rolling an odd number, and then the probability that it greater than three *given* it is odd. We may now consider these two probabilities as independent, thus they may be multiplied together to produce a probability for the joint event of a single die roll producing an outcome which is an odd number, and, greater than three. This is $1/2 \times 1/3 = 1/6$ which, as might be expected, is the same as when we considered the outcome by enumeration above.

Generally we can say that:

$$Pr(A, B) = Pr(A) \times Pr(B|A) \tag{2}$$

This is known as the *third law of probability for dependent events* where A and B can have the same meaning as in the example above and the symbol | means *given*. In the case above $Pr(B|A)$ meant the probability that a number was odd *given* it was greater than three. There were three possible outcomes greater than 3, only one of which was odd, so $Pr(B|A) = 1/3$.

This version of the *third law* is more general, and consequently more important than the version of the *third law of probability* which assumes independence between events. It features prominently in evidence evaluation, and will be referred to later in this book (See Appendix H).

3.2 Binomial probability

In Section 2.3 we examined the distribution of THC content of marijuana by arranging the measured THC from sample of observations from 1986 seizures into groups of ascending order. Here we return to the idea of distribution, but rather than thinking of a distribution as something which is purely measured, distributions for certain events can be calculated from theory.

Consider the model of coin throwing. If a fair coin is tossed then it has two sides, and the probability of throwing a head is $Pr(H) = 1/2 = 0.5$, which is also the probability of throwing a tail. If the coin is thrown twice then the joint event of throwing a head followed by a tail from Section 3.1 is $Pr(H, T) = 1/2 \times 1/2 = 1/4 = 0.25$, which is also the probability of throwing a tail followed by a head and the probability of two tails, or two heads.

However, what we are now interested in are the counts of heads and tails regardless of the ordering for a given number of throws of the coin. In the example above for two throws of the coin the probability of throwing two heads is $1/4$, and the probability of two tails is also $1/4$. The probability of throwing a head followed by a tail is $1/4$ as is the probability of throwing a tail followed by a head. If the ordering is unimportant and we are looking only at numbers of heads and tails for two throws, then the event of throwing a head followed by a tail is the same as throwing a tail followed by a head. Each involves throwing one head and one tail, but there are two ways of doing this, so the probability of throwing one head and one tail from two throws of the dice is $1/4 + 1/4 = 1/2$.

If a fair coin is now tossed three times we know that there are $2 \times 2 \times 2 = 2^3 = 8$ possible outcomes. These are exhaustively enumerated in Figure 3.1.

Table 3.1 gives the occurrence of 0 heads, 1 head and so on from the tree diagram in Figure 3.1, and are simply counted from the furthest right column of the table. The

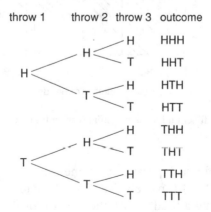

Figure 3.1 Tree diagram showing every possible outcome for three throws of a (fair) coin

Table 3.1   Probabilities for all possible outcomes for tossing a
fair coin three times

Number of heads	0	1	2	3
Number of tails	3	2	1	0
Occurrences	1	3	3	1
Probability	1/8	3/8	3/8	1/8

probability of each result from three tosses is simply the number of ways in which
the outcome can occur divided by the total numbers of equally likely outcomes. In
this case the total number of outcomes is eight. So, for instance, there is only one
way in which three heads can be obtained from three tosses of the coin, that is HHH,
there are eight equally likely outcomes, so the probability of having three heads from
three coin tosses is 1/8. There are three ways of having a single head from three
coin tosses, namely HTT, THT, and TTH, so there is a 3/8 probability of obtaining
a single head from three tosses.

The row marked 'probability' from Table 3.1 is known as a probability density
function. In this case it is a *binomial distribution* for the range 0 to 3 with probability
of each event as 1/2. A graph of it can be drawn as in Figure 3.2.

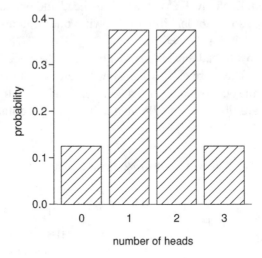

Figure 3.2   Probability function for the binomial distribution with three trials and a probability
of 1/2

The probabilities for each possible outcome can be read from the graph in the
same way as from Table 3.1, namely that, from three tosses of a coin for which the
probability of throwing a head is 1/2, there is a probability of 1/8 of getting no
heads, 3/8 of throwing one or two heads, and a probability of 1/8 that both tosses
result in a head.

We do not have to draw a diagram to enumerate all possible outcomes as we have done in Figure 3.1. We can just calculate the probabilities we wish to know from the formula for a binomial probability. The equation for a binomial probability is:

$$Pr(X = x) = \frac{n!}{x!(n-x)!} \; p^x(1-p)^{(n-x)} \tag{3}$$

Where:

n number of trials – in the case above it is three.

x the number of outcomes of the particular value for which we are calculating the probability.

p the probability of the outcome, in the case above it is 1/2.

$x!$ denotes the factorial expansion; e.g. $x! = x \times (x-1) \times \ldots 2 \times 1$; $5! = 5 \times 4 \times 3 \times 2 \times 1 = 120$

For example, in the first instance, where we calculate the probability of throwing 0 heads, we substitute the value 0 in for x, 3 in for n and 1/2 in for p. This gives:

$$Pr(x = 0) = \frac{3!}{0!(3-0)!} (1/2)^0 (1-(1/2))^{(3-0)}$$

$$= \frac{3 \times 2 \times 1}{1 \times 3 \times 2 \times 1} \times 1 \times (1/2)^3$$

$$= 1 \times 1 \times (1/2)^3$$

$$= 1/8$$

by substituting[‡] into Equation 3, 1 for x, n remaining equal to 3 and p to 1/2 the probability of finding one head in a series of three tosses can be calculated:

$$Pr(x = 1) = \frac{3!}{1!(3-1)!} (1/2)^1 (1-(1/2))^{(3-1)}$$

$$= \frac{3 \times 2 \times 1}{1 \times 2 \times 1} \times (1/2) \times (1/2)^2$$

$$= 3 \times (1/2) \times (1/2)^2$$

$$= 3/8.$$

From this the probabilities for each possible set of outcomes from the throwing of three coins can be calculated.

Obviously, the binomial distribution is not restricted to probabilities of 1/2 and small numbers for n. If the proportion of red cars on Britain's roads were 1/10 it would be possible to calculate the probability of seeing exactly 15 red cars in a car

---

[‡] Note: $0! = 1$

park of 200 randomly parked cars by substituting $x = 15$, $n = 200$ and $p = 1/10$ into Equation 3. This would be:

$$\Pr(x = 15) = \frac{200!}{15!(200 - 15)!} (1/10)^{15}(1 - (1/10))^{(200-15)}$$

$$= \frac{200!}{15!185!} \times (1/10)^{15} \times (9/10)^{185}$$

$$= \frac{200 \times 199 \times 198 \times \ldots \times 188 \times 187 \times 186}{15!}$$

$$(1/10)^{15} \times (9/10)^{185}$$

$$= 1.463 \times 10^{22} \times 1 \times 10^{-15} \times 3.427 \times 10^{-9}$$

$$= 0.0501$$

or just over 5%.

3.3 Poisson probability

Calculating the binomial probability for the observation of 15 red cars in a car park of some 200 cars is quite difficult as there are many factorial expansions to calculate. For large numbers such as 200, even a modern computer has some difficulty. An approximation to a binomial probability is a Poisson probability, and is a good approximation to a binomial probability for these sorts of large number where the event of interest occurs with a low probability.

The probability function for a Poisson probability is:

$$\Pr(X = x) = \frac{\lambda^x e^{-\lambda}}{x!} \tag{4}$$

where x is the same as for binomial probabilities, and is the number of outcomes in which we have a particular interest, and λ is the expected frequency of the outcomes of particular interest. Thus, in the example above we are interested in the probability of seeing 15 red cars in a car park containing 200 cars, so x is 15. As red cars occur with a probability of $1/10$ we expect to see $1/10 \times 200 = 20$ from a sample of 200 cars. Substituting these values into Equation 4 we find:

$$\Pr(X = 15) = \frac{20^{15} \ e^{-20}}{15!}$$

$$= \frac{3.27 \times 10^{19} \times 2.06 \times 10^{-9}}{1.30 \times 10^{12}}$$

$$= 0.0518$$

which is a good approximation to 0.0501 calculated from Equation 3 above.

A useful feature of the Poisson is that there is no need to specify a sample size as long as an expected frequency can be calculated for the number of events observed.

This is useful where we may wish to calculate the probabilities for events which are rare compared with a large potential sample size. This could arise where a particular facet of an individual, say a particular genotype, might be expected to occur only five times in the population of the United Kingdom. It may be expected to occur only five times in the population, but there is a probability it will not occur at all, or occur only once. Using a binomial probability for these events would be extremely difficult as the population of the United Kingdom is about 60 million, and the factorial expansion of 60 million is incalculably large. However, using a Poisson approximation to a binomial probability the calculations become relatively simple. Substituting 0 for x, and 5 for λ into Equation 4:

$$\Pr(X = 0) = \frac{5^0 \times e^{-5}}{0!}$$
$$= \frac{1 \times 0.0067}{1}$$
$$= 0.0067$$

which is the probability of observing 0 individuals with the particular genotype in the United Kingdom.

3.4 Empirical probability

In contrast to the aleatory situation where a model is fully understood in terms of a physical structure, as in coins, dice, or cards, one can look at probabilities from an *empirical* stance as we did with THC in marijuana in Section 2.3. This is much more useful in forensic science where very few problems involve the random systems of the dice game, and involves observing and measuring properties of entities in the world around us. The presumption is that there is some underlying feature or principle of the world which makes the observations of the entities in it take on the form they do. The point of many sciences is to use these observations to work back to the laws which form the empirical observations using the principles of probability deduced from aleatory systems, rather than start with the underlying mechanics for a full description of the system. This approach has its problems. Observations are usually based on samples, so uncertainty pervades every aspect of the study. However, the same principles of probability seen in aleatory systems can be used, using the same mathematical principles, in subject areas which use empirical data.

Modelling empirical probabilities

There are circumstances where, based upon some summary statistic and our knowledge of some underlying distribution, probabilities for a range of outcomes can be calculated. This process is called modelling, and rather than taking an aleatory probability from a known system, the probability can be supplied through observation. For example, a brief survey of 135 men in the mathematics and physics departments of Edinburgh University indicated that 25 of the male population had either a beard and/or moustache, therefore the probability of finding a male with a beard and/or moustache amongst this group is $25/135 = 0.185$.

If this frequency of beards and/or moustaches is reflected in the population of men as a whole, then in a sample of 25 men randomly drawn from the population, the probability distribution for the number of men with a beard and/or moustache can be modelled by calculating binomial probabilities for each possible outcome in exactly the same way that we did earlier for three tosses of a coin. Only this time we calculate binomial probabilities from 0 to 25 using Equation 3 with a probability of 0.185. This distribution is given in Figure 3.3.

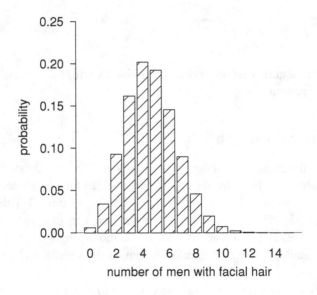

Figure 3.3 Probability function for the binomial distribution with 25 trials and a probability of 0.185. Only $x \leq 15$ is given for clarity as when $x > 15$ $Pr(X = x) \approx 0$

The data from Figure 3.3 is also given in table form as Table 3.2.

The modal probability is about four males with a beard and/or moustache from the sample of 25 males as 18.5% of 25 is 4.6.

However, we can also frame different questions. For example, the probability of finding five or fewer males with a beard and/or moustache can be treated in the same way as getting a two or three from a throw of a fair dice. Using the second law of probability we can add the probabilities of all the outcomes which fit the criteria. In the instance of an outcome of five or fewer males with beards and/or moustaches from a sample of 25 would be $0.006 + 0.034 + 0.093 + 0.162 + 0.202 + 0.192 = 0.689$. This means that were one to inspect 25 males there would be a 68.9% probability that fewer than six would have a beard and/or moustache.

Table 3.2 The probabilities of observing 0 to 25 men who possess a beard/moustach from a sample of 25 men it the probability of each man possessing a beard/moustach is 0.185.

Men	Probability
0	0.006
1	0.034
2	0.093
3	0.162
4	0.202
5	0.192
6	0.146
7	0.090
8	0.046
9	0.020
10	0.007
11	0.002
12	0.001
≥ 13	0.000

Truly empirical probabilities

If we have data we do not always need to have a precise model to be able to make the same type of inferences about outcomes. For instance the data from THC content from Section 2.2 can also be treated as a probability function. All we have to do is take the frequencies seen in THC content in seizures from 1986 (Figure 1.1), and divide each frequency in each THC category by the sum of all the frequencies and we have an empirical probability function. This is shown in Figure 3.4.

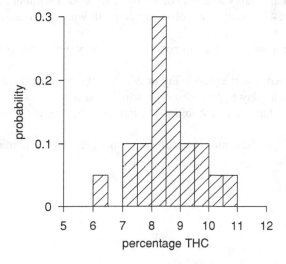

Figure 3.4 Empirical probability function for the THC content of marijuana from 1986

Table 3.3   Empirical probability density for
the THC content of sample marijuana from
1986 calculated from the counts in Figure 1.1

$\Delta^9 - THC(\%)$	Counts	Probability
6.0 → 6.5	1	0.05
6.5 → 7.0	0	0.00
7.0 → 7.5	2	0.10
7.5 → 8.0	2	0.10
8.0 → 8.5	6	0.30
8.5 → 9.0	3	0.15
9.0 → 9.5	2	0.10
9.5 → 10.0	2	0.10
10.0 → 10.5	1	0.05
10.5 → 11.0	1	0.05

The values for the probability density function from Figure 3.4 are given in Table 3.3.

This can be used in exactly the same way as the binomial probability density function for men with beards and/or moustaches from a sample of 25 men seen in Figure 3.3. For example, using the second law of probability, the probability that any marijuana from 1986 has a THC content greater than 10% is $0.05 + 0.05 = 0.1$ or 1%. The probability that marijuana from 1986 has a THC content between 7% and 10% can be calculated as $0.10 + 0.10 + 0.30 + 0.15 + 0.10 + 0.10 = 0.85$, or 85%.

Review questions

1. In the National Lottery a sample of six balls are drawn without replacement from a population of 49, what is the probability you will win with five tickets?

2. What is the probability you will not win the Lottery with your five tickets?

3. Having decided that the probability of winning the National Lottery is too low you have decided to play a game of dice in which you win if you score three sixes from five throws. What is the probability of winning? The dice is fair and six sided.

4. Use Table 3.3 to determine the probability that the THC content of marijuana from 1986 is $\leq 8\%$.

4 The normal distribution

In Section 3.2 we saw how the binomial distribution could be used to calculate probabilities for specific outcomes for runs of events based upon either a known probability, or an observed probability, for a single event. We also saw how an empirical probability distribution can be treated in exactly the same way as a modelled distribution. Both these distributions were for discrete data types, or for continuous types made into discrete data. In this section we deal with the normal distribution, which is a probability distribution applied to continuous data.

4.1 The normal distribution

The normal distribution[†] is possibly the most commonly used continuous distribution in statistical science. This is because it is a theoretically appealing model to explain many forms of natural continuous variation. Many of the discrete distributions may be approximated by the normal distribution for large samples. Most continuous variables, particularly from biological sciences, are distributed normally, or can be transformed to a normal distribution.

Imagine a continuous random variable such as the length of the femur in adult humans. The mean length of this bone is about 400 mm, some are 450 mm and some are 350 mm, but there are not many in either of these categories. If the distribution is plotted then we expect to see a shape with its maximum height at about 400 mm tailing off to either side. These shapes have been plotted for both the adult human femur and adult human tibia in Figure 4.1.

The tibia in any individual is usually shorter than the femur, however, Figure 4.1 tells us that some people have tibias which are longer than other people's femurs. Notice how the mean of tibia measurements is shorter than the mean of the femur

[†] Often called the Gaussian distribution.

Introduction to Statistics for Forensic Scientists   David Lucy
© 2005 John Wiley & Sons, Ltd.

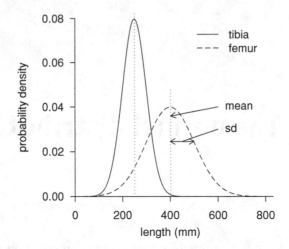

Figure 4.1 Probability density functions (PDF) for adult human femurs and tibias. The mean and standard deviation of the femur PDF are arrowed

measurements. Also how the femurs are more spread out than the tibias, leading the probability density function for the tibias to be more peaked than that for the femurs.

Each of the normal distributions in Figure 4.1 has two *parameters* which control what it looks like. First, there is the mean which is the location about which the distribution is centred; for the tibias this is 250 mm, for the femurs this is 400 mm. Secondly, there is the dispersion parameter called the standard deviation, the larger the standard deviation the lower the peak at the mean, the smaller the standard deviation the more pointed the distribution appears. This can be seen in Figure 4.1 where the tibia distribution is more peaked than that for the femurs, this is because the distribution for femurs has a larger standard deviation than that for tibias.

4.2 Standard deviation and standard error of the mean

It happens that because we imagine that variables distributed with random error are somehow manifestations of an underlying normal distribution we can use data from a sample to calculate what that normal distribution is like. This process is another example of *modelling* because we are now assuming, perhaps with good reason, that the real distribution of the population from which the sample is taken is normal.

From Section 4 we know that the normal distribution has a mean, and a standard deviation. These are called *parameters*, and any analysis using distributional assumptions is generally termed *parametric statistics*. Parameters are denoted by Greek letters such as μ or θ for the mean, and σ^2 for the variance. Estimates are denoted by Roman letters such as $\bar{x}$ for the mean and s^2 for the variance. Sometimes estimates are denoted with a *hat* over the parameter symbol. Thus $\hat{\theta}$ for an estimate of the mean, and $\hat{\sigma}^2$ for the variance.

The sample standard deviation is defined as the square root of the sample variance, that is:

$$\text{variance } (x) = \frac{\sum_{i=1}^{n}(x_i - \overline{x})^2}{n - 1} \tag{5}$$

therefore:

$$\text{standard deviation } (x) = \sqrt{\frac{\sum_{i=1}^{n}(x_i - \overline{x})^2}{n - 1}} \tag{6}$$

For the array ($x = \{2, 4, 3, 5, 4\}$) the variance (see Section 2.5) is $(2.56 + 0.16 + 0.36 + 1.96 + 0.16)/(5 - 1) = 1.3$, so the standard deviation (sd) is $\sqrt{1.3} = 1.14$. The array $x = \{2, 4, 3, 5, 4\}$ can be considered to be a sample from a distribution with unknown mean, estimated by $\overline{x} = 3.6$, and standard deviation, estimated by $s = 1.14$.

There is another measure sometimes referred to in the literature, that is the *standard error of the mean*, or more simply the *standard error*. This is not to be confused with the standard deviation, and arises from the fact that $\overline{x}$ is an estimate of the mean. Because $\overline{x}$ is an estimate uncertainty is associated with different samples from the same population. Were we repeatedly to sample from the same population the means of the samples would be unlikely to be the same in each case. This means that our estimates of the population mean would also vary. This variability is called the standard error of the mean. The standard error of the mean (se) is calculated by dividing the standard deviation by $\sqrt{n}$, so:

$$\text{standard error of the mean } (x) = \frac{\text{sd}}{\sqrt{n}} \tag{7}$$

In the example above the sd is 1.14, so the se is $1.14/\sqrt{5} = 1.14/2.24 = 0.51$.

Figure 4.2 shows the THC concentrations in marijuana concentrations in Figure 4.1 with the normal model superimposed. The model has been calculated from the data in Section 2.1, and from Section 2.4 has a mean of 8.59, the variance is 1.19, hence the sd is 1.09.

The sample size (n) of the THC samples from 1986 is 20, so the standard error of the mean is $1.09/\sqrt{20} = 0.24$. Notice that were n equal to a lower number, say 6, then if the variance remained unchanged but the standard error would be $1.09/\sqrt{6} = 0.45$, which is larger than with $n = 20$. This is a measure of the precision with which the population mean is estimated by the sample mean. The smaller the standard error the greater the precision of the estimate[‡].

[‡] For instance, were one to double the precision then one must use a sample size of four times that used initially.

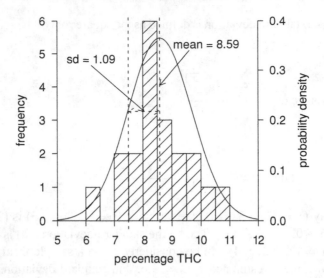

Figure 4.2 Probability density function superimposed on the histogram (as in Figure 4.1) of Δ^9-THC concentration in marijuana seizures from 1986. Marked on the normal curve is the mean and the standard deviation

4.3 Percentage points of the normal distribution

In Section 3.4 we used an empirical probability density function to calculate the probability of finding five or fewer males with beards or moustaches from a sample of 25 males, given that 18.5% of the male population has a beard (it was 68.9%). This was done by summing the probabilities of finding 0 or 1 or 2 or ... 5 males from the same sample. Very much the same thing can be done with the normal distribution, only the summation has to be calculated using a mathematical process called integration. As integration is a difficult process statisticians have calculated tables for a standardized normal distribution which can be rescaled to fit any particular normal distribution. This result of this standardization is called the *standard normal distribution*, and it has a mean of 0 and standard deviation of 1. Figure 4.3 shows the standard normal distribution, and Appendix B is such a table of summed areas at each point for the standard normal distribution.

The shaded area under the standard normal curve extends from $-\infty^\S$ to two standard deviations. In fact it is the same diagram as in the top right corner of Appendix B. If we wish to find the area under this portion of the curve we simply look down the rows of Appendix B until we reach the row labelled $z = 2.0^\P$. For the third decimal place the appropriate column is selected. In the case of 2 standard

---

§ ∞ is notation for infinity, the normal distribution is asymptotic in that it goes from $-\infty$ to ∞, so values occurring at very large $-$ve or $+$ve values of the standard deviation are not impossible, however they are extremely unlikely. The probability density in any of the tails never reaches zero.
¶ Standardized variables obtained by subtracting the mean and dividing the result by the standard deviation are sometimes referred to as z-scores, or z for short.

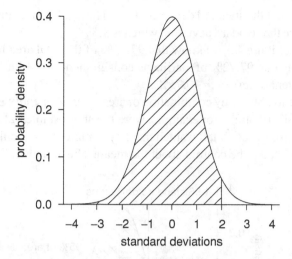

Figure 4.3   Standard normal distribution with mean 0 and standard deviation equal to 1. The shaded area covers the range $-\infty$ to 2 standard deviations

deviations it is the first column, which has the value 0.9772. As the standard normal distribution is a probability distribution the total area under the curve must equal 1, so the value 0.9772 means that 97.72% of the total area, hence probability for the distribution, lies between $-\infty$ and 2 standard deviations.

Figure 4.4 is the same distribution shown in Figure 4.3 but rescaled to the normal distribution underlying the Δ^9-THC content sample from 1986. In this case the

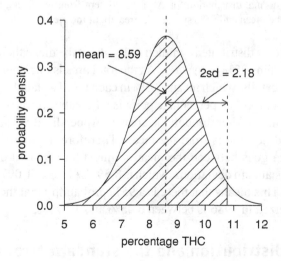

Figure 4.4   The normal distribution for Δ^9-THC content from marijuana consignments seized in 1986. This the same distribution as that depicted in Figure 4.2, and has mean 8.59 and standard deviation 1.09. The shaded area covers the range $-\infty$ to 2 standard deviations which occurs at $8.59 + (2 \times 1.09) = 10.77\%$

mean is 8.59% and the standard deviation 1.09. The shaded area upper limit is at the mean plus twice the standard deviation which is $8.59 + (2 \times 1.09) = 8.59 + 2.16 = 10.75$. As from Figure 4.3 we know that 97.72% of the total area lies in the shaded zone we can say that 97.72% of marijuana consignments seized in 1986 will have a morphene content of *less than* 10.75%.

It is possible to obtain any combination of areas from Appendix B and apply them to any normal distribution. For example, were the shortest interval in which 95% of THC samples from 1986 to fall wanted then, by symmetry, we could start by saying that the interval had to be centred about the mean. This is shown in Figure 4.5.

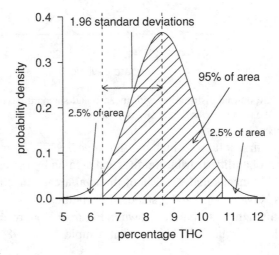

Figure 4.5   The normal distribution for Δ^9-THC content from marijuana consignments seized in 1986 showing the mean and 95% symmetric area about the mean

As 95% has to be distributed symmetrically about the mean then we know that the shaded area contains 95% of the area. As the total area is one, there has to be 5% for the total over both tails, which means 2.5% in each tail. The tabulation in Appendix B means that the appropriate percentage point is where the area is 97.50%, as we want 2.5% in each tail. Looking through the areas in Appendix B we see that 0.9750 lies at 1.96 standard deviations from the mean. Therefore the interval which contains 95% of the area goes between the mean minus 1.96 standard deviations and the mean plus 1.96 standard deviations, which is $8.59 \pm (1.96 \times 1.09) = 8.59 \pm 2.13 = 6.45 \rightarrow 10.73$. This means that there is a 95% probability that the Δ^9-THC content of marijuana seized in 1986 is between 6.45% and 10.73%.

4.4 The *t*-distribution and the standard error of the mean

The standard error of the mean as given in Section 4.2 is given as the standard deviation divided by the square root of the sample size. It is a measure of the spread of confidence for the population mean when it has been estimated by the mean of a sample taken from the population. For instance, for the Δ^9-THC concentration in marijuana from 1986 the standard deviation is 1.09%, so the standard error for a sample size of 20 for the estimate of the mean is $1.09/4.47 = 0.244\%$.

A mean, however, is not in itself distributed with a normal distribution. When we talk about means and differences between means we tend to think in terms of a *t-distribution*. The *t*-distribution is rather like the normal distribution in that it is another symmetric unimodal distribution. The *t*-distribution has only one parameter defining its shape. This parameter is called the *degrees of freedom* (df), and is based on the sample size.

Figure 4.6 shows a *t*-distribution with df = 4. Superimposed is a standard normal. The two tails of the *t*-distribution are shaded, each containing 2.5% of the total area, consequently 95% remains unshaded. From Figure 4.6 it can be seen that the *t*-distribution is less pointed than the standard normal, however, as the degrees of freedom (the parameter of the *t*-distribution) increase it gradually takes on the shape of the normal. In fact at df = ∞ the *t*-distribution is exactly the same as a normal.

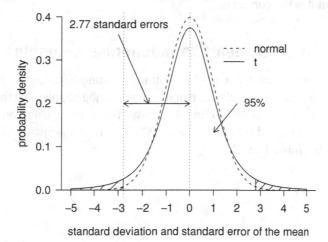

standard deviation and standard error of the mean

Figure 4.6 *t*-distribution (df = 4) with a standard normal superimposed, the tails for the *t*-distribution are shaded and contain 2.5% of the area in each

The *t*-distribution may be used to estimate a confidence interval for the population mean when the variance of the population is estimated from a sample. From above the estimate of mean concentration of Δ^9-THC in marijuana seizures from 1986 is 8.59%, but as that is a figure based on a sample of 20 there is some uncertainty associated with it. To calculate a 95% confidence interval for the mean we first need the number of standard errors which enclose 95% of the area of the *t*-distribution for df = 19[||]. Appendix C has these tabulated. Essentially look down column 1

[||] The degrees of freedom are the number of measurements which are allowed to vary. So if I have a sequence of five non-negative integers which add up to, say 13, then the first four can be any numbers between 0 and 13, however, the last number is determined by the constraint of adding up to 13, so there are $5 - 1 = 4$ degrees of freedom in this case.

until df $= 19$ is found, and at 5% (in both tails) this is at 2.093 standard errors. We can say from this that the 95% confidence interval is the mean ± 2.093 standard errors $= 8.59 \pm 2.093 \times 0.244 = 8.59 \pm 0.510 = 8.08 \rightarrow 9.10$. This is interpreted that there is a 95% confidence that the true mean Δ^9-THC content of marijuana from 1986 seizures is between 8.08% and 9.10%.

Using the example above, were a 99% confidence region for the mean to be required the second column of Appendix C would be used. The mean is again 8.59% the standard error of the mean 0.244 but the confidence region is of width 2.861 standard errors. This would give $8.59 \pm (0.244 \times 2.861) = 8.59 \pm 0.698$, so there would be a 99% confidence that the mean Δ^9-THC concentration of marijuana from 1986 is between 7.89% and 9.29%.

This calculated confidence should *not* be interpreted as a probability distribution for the mean of the population based on the sample. It is the interval where 99% of means from different samples of the same population would fall given a sufficiently long run of sampling. This definition may seem to be unusually stringent and pedantic, but it is the correct one.

4.5 *t*-testing between two independent samples

A more widespread use for the *t*-distribution is testing between the means of two samples to examine the hypotheses that the means of the populations from which the samples are drawn are equal. Figure 4.7 shows two such distributions which have been randomly sampled from the data on Δ^9-THC from marijuana seizures during 1986 (See also Table 4.1).

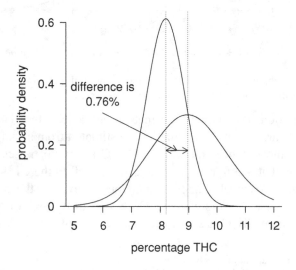

Figure 4.7   Normal models for two sub-samples of $n = 10$ for the Δ^9-THC from seizures during 1986

Table 4.1   Summary statistics for two sub-samples of Δ^9-THC from seizures during 1986 from Figure 4.4

Subsample	n_i	Mean	Variance	sd	se Mean
1	10	8.968%	1.763	1.327	0.134
2	10	8.203%	0.424	0.651	0.557

From Figure 4.7 even random sampling from the same set of data has, in this instance, led to a difference in the means of the two sub-samples of 0.76%. The object of a *t*-test is to look at the differences in means and see whether the difference is due to chance selection, or some real populational difference.

Conventionally we start by erecting two hypotheses. The *null* hypothesis, usually denoted H_0, is one of no difference, or that the means of the two sub-samples can be regarded as being selected from the same population. The second hypothesis is complementary to the *null* hypothesis and is called the *alternative* hypothesis, denoted H_1. It states that the means from the two sub-samples are *not* equal, and that there are grounds for treating the two sub-samples as being drawn from different populations.

The difference in the mean values of sub-sample 1 and sub-sample 2 is 0.77%, and this difference will have a distribution centred around 0.77% with a dispersion $(se(x_1 - x_2))$ given by:

$$se(x_1 - x_2) = \hat{s}\sqrt{\frac{1}{n_1} + \frac{1}{n_2}} \tag{8}$$

where:

x_1 sub-sample 1
x_2 sub-sample 2
n_1 *n* for sub-sample 1
n_2 *n* for sub-sample 2

The term $\hat{s}$ on the right-hand side of the equation is an estimate for the *pooled* variance. The reason we need a pooled variance is that we are trying to estimate a distribution for the difference between the two means. We cannot have a single unimodal distribution which has two variances, so we need a single estimate of variance. This is done by a form of weighted average of the two component variances given by:

$$\hat{s} = \sqrt{\frac{(n_1 - 1)s_1^2 + (n_2 - 1)s_2^2}{n_1 + n_2 - 2}} \tag{9}$$

where s_1^2 and s_2^2 are the *variances* of the two subsamples. Substituting the information in Table 4.5 into Equation 9:

$$\hat{s} = \sqrt{\frac{(9 \times 1.76) + (9 \times 0.42)}{9 + 9 - 2}}$$

$$= \sqrt{\frac{15.87 + 3.82}{16}}$$

$$= 1.11$$

Taking the estimate of $\hat{s}$ and substituting into Equation 8:

$$se(x_1 - x_2) = 1.11\sqrt{\frac{1}{10} + \frac{1}{10}}$$

$$= 1.11\sqrt{\frac{1}{5}}$$

$$= 0.50.$$

The estimate of the standard error for the *difference* between the two sample means is 0.50%. From Appendix C 95% of the probability for the difference between the two sample means will lie within 2.101[**] standard errors of the mean, so a confidence interval for the *difference* of 0.76% will be 0.76% $\pm (0.50 \times 2.101) = 0.76 \pm 1.05$ thus the confidence interval is $-0.29 \rightarrow 1.81$.

The 95% confidence interval contains zero as a possible value for the difference in means between the two samples. Hence one would accept the hypothesis (H_0), conclude that there is no statistically significant difference in the means of the subsamples at 95% confidence (or 5% significance), and these samples could have been taken from consignments with the same mean THC content.

The Δ^9-THC contents for seizures from 1986 and 1987 can both be modelled by normal distributions. Figure 4.8 shows these models. Summary statistics appear in Table 4.2.

Substituting information from Table 4.2 into Equation 9:

$$\hat{s} = \sqrt{\frac{(19 \times 1.19) + (14 \times 0.39)}{20 + 15 - 2}}$$

$$= \sqrt{\frac{22.61 + 5.46}{33}}$$

$$= 0.92$$

[**]This is another degrees of freedom where for a two sample t-test one uses $n_1 + n_2 - 2$ df, which will be in column 1 of Appendix C.

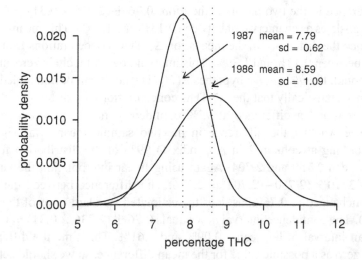

Figure 4.8 Normal models for Δ-THC concentrations from marijuana seizures from 1986 and 1987. The parameters are taken the values in Table 2.2 and are based on sample sizes of 20 from 1986 and 15 from 1987. The means are indicated by dotted vertical lines.

Table 4.2 Summary statistics THC concentrations in marijuana from 1986 and 1987 seizures from Figure 4.8

Seizure date	n_i	Mean	Variance	sd	se Mean
1986	20	8.59%	1.19	1.09	0.24
1987	15	7.79%	0.39	0.62	0.16

and $\hat{s}$ into Equation 8:

$$se(x_1 - x_2) = 0.92\sqrt{\frac{1}{20} + \frac{1}{15}}$$

$$= 0.92\sqrt{\frac{7}{60}}$$

$$= 0.31$$

The difference in the two means is $8.58 - 7.79 = 0.76\%$, with dispersion distributed t with 33 df, and standard error 0.31. Looking at Appendix C we see that there is no specific value for a t with 33 df, instead we have df $= 30$ and df $= 40$. The solution is simply to add 3/10ths of the difference to the lower of the two (one could equally remove 7/10ths of the difference from the upper). The difference from Appendix C is $2.042 - 2.021 = 0.021$; 3/10ths $\times 0.021 = 0.0063$, so the value of t is $2.042 - 0.0063 = 2.036$ standard errors[††]. A 95% confidence interval for

[††]This process is called linear interpolation. More accurate values can be obtained from computer software.

the difference in the two means is therefore $0.76 \pm (2.036 \times 0.31) = 0.76 \pm 0.63$ which translates as an interval of between 0.13% and 1.39%. This means that at 95% confidence the difference in the means for Δ^9-THC concentrations from 1986 and 1987 is between 0.13% and 1.39%. This interval does not include zero, and we may act as though the *alternative* hypothesis (H_1) is true. It can be concluded with 95% confidence statistically that the Δ^9-THC concentrations are different.

Having found a difference at 95% confidence interval it would be interesting to see whether the difference in the two sample means was significant at 99%. Looking at column 2 in Appendix D 99% of the distribution for df $= 33$ falls between 2.750 and 2.704. Again using linear interpolation the value of t is $2.750 - 3/10 \times (2.750 - 2.704) = 2.736$. The difference between the means remains unchanged at 0.76%, as does the estimated standard error of the difference (0.31%). The confidence interval now equals $0.76 \pm (2.736 \times 0.31) = 0.76 \pm 0.85$ giving an interval of between -0.09% and 1.61%. This time the difference does include zero as a possible value for the mean difference, so we should act as though the hypothesis (H_0) were true. It should be concluded that at 99% confidence the difference in Δ^9-THC concentration between marijuana seized in 1986 and 1987 is not statistically significant.

Correct statistical interpretation of these confidence intervals is critical. A 95% confidence interval means that in a 'long run' of sampling and comparison 95% of the differences in means between the two samples would lie within the confidence interval. It does *not* mean that there is a 95% chance that the *null hypothesis*, if accepted, is correct, or that there is a 95% chance that the *alternative hypothesis* is correct, if that is accepted. See Section 4.7 for a fuller discussion of the statistical interpretation of the terms confidence and significance.

4.6 Testing between paired observations

Sometimes a question will arise concerning the differences between two means which may not be considered independent. A typical application is where two different treatments are applied to the same sample of individuals so that each individual receives treatment A, then treatment B, some observations of interest being taken for each individual under each treatment.

Here, because each treatment has not been applied to separate samples selected randomly from some wider population, we could expect that the observations are going to be dependent on each other. The way in which this is dealt with is to look at the distribution of differences between treatment A and treatment B. If the effects of treatment A are equivalent to the effects of treatment B then the mean of the differences should be equal to zero. Of course, because the observations are subject to uncertainty it would be unusual for the differences to be exactly zero were there no differences between treatment A and B. So we need to define precisely how large the mean of differences should be before thinking that there is a real effect between the two treatments.

To illustrate this procedure we can look at the work of Martin *et al.* (In press) which examined the effect of using phosphate buffered solution (PBS) and water on the number of cells extracted from swabs taken from each of three occasions from six different donors. Table 4.3 gives the number of cells observed after extraction under the two treatments for their sample of men.

Table 4.3   Number of cells recovered from swabs from men under two different extraction regimes, water and phosphate buffered solution reproduced with permission.

Donor	Occasion	no. cells Water	no. cells PBS
1	1	354	1623
1	2	318	535
1	3	1031	681
2	1	453	847
2	2	960	1987
2	3	531	1078
3	1	3021	1595
3	2	2840	6998
3	3	4820	5410

If, for the data in Table 4.3, we are prepared to consider each different occasion for each different donor as independent the effects of water and PBS can be examined using a one sample *t*-test.

Table 4.4 gives the mean difference between extraction in water and PBS as -714 cells, the larger mean being for the PBS extraction medium. Is this difference significant though? Were the two extraction methods to yield the same number of cells then we would expect this difference to be zero, so could it be that a difference of -714 cells is indistinguishable from a difference of zero?

Table 4.4   Means and differences of numbers of cells from three men on each of three occasions

Cells water (x_1)	Cells PBS (x_1)	Difference (d)	$d - \bar{d}$	$(d - \bar{d})^2$
354	1623	-1269	-555	308025
318	535	-217	497	247009
1031	681	350	1064	1132096
453	847	-394	320	102400
960	1987	-1027	-313	97969
531	1078	-547	167	27889
3021	1595	1426	2140	4579600
2840	6998	-4158	-3444	11861136
4820	5410	-590	124	15376
$\bar{x}_1 = 1592$	$\bar{x}_2 = 2306$	$\bar{d} = -714$		$\sum = 18371500$

The sum of squared deviations (column 5, Table 4.4) is 18371500, so the variance is $18371500/(n-1) = 2296438$. The standard deviation is the square root of the variance, so is $\sqrt{2296438} = 1515.4$. The standard error of the mean is the standard error divided by the square root of n which, in this case, is $1515.4/\sqrt{9} = 1515.4/3 = 505.13$.

A 95% confidence interval for the mean of -714 cells can be calculated from the standard error (above) and from the tabulated value of t for $n - 1 = 8$ degrees of freedom in Appendix C. This value of t is 2.306, so a 95% confidence interval for the mean difference is $-714 \pm (2.306 \times 505.13) = 714 \pm 1164.8$, or, $-1878.84 \rightarrow 450.84$. This confidence interval includes zero, so at 95% confidence zero is a possible value for the mean difference. This gives us grounds for accepting the null hypothesis, and acting as though there were no differences in the incidence of cell recovery between water and PBS. The same comments apply to the statistical interpretation of the confidence interval as in the two sample case above.

It should be noted that here we have an ordinal variable, number of cells, being transposed to a categorical variable. This is possible if the ordinal variable has a sufficient number of separate levels. In this case we can see from Table 4.3 that the number of cells has a range from 535 to 5410 giving at least 4875 separate levels, which is perfectly reasonable number to warrant treatment of the variable as continuous.

4.7 Confidence, significance and p-values

The testing type statistics which we have seen above are all classical frequentist tests. Some points, notably looking at percentage points of the normal distribution for Δ^9-THC to determine probabilities, have been given a Bayesian interpretation without much thought to the exact nature of that probability. However to understand the t-tests and other classical hypothesis tests it is necessary to consider exactly what is meant by the various terms used.

The *null* hypothesis, conventionally denoted H_0, in terms of t-testing is a hypothesis which suggests there be no differences in the means of the two samples, or in the one sample test the differences in measurements are equal to zero. Complementary to the *null* hypothesis is the *alternative* hypothesis which is a hypothesis of difference. In some tests, such as the two sample t-test, this would indicate that the sample means were different, or that the differences in measurements were not equal to zero in the one sample case, were the alternative hypothesis true.

In hypothesis testing we calculate the differences in respect of some distribution and see whether those differences are greater, or less than, some predefined point conventionally denoted as α, to which we will return. If the differences are greater than a quantity suggested by α we act as though H_0 were false, and we accept H_1. If the observed differences are less we act as though H_0 were true.

Of course, data are always variable, and we cannot know for sure whether, on the basis of any test, we have made the correct decision. What we can do is to calculate the probability that we have made the right decision.

For any test with mutually exclusive and exhaustive binary outcomes there are two potential outcomes, and two potential 'truths'. Therefore there are four possibilities. We can get it right by accepting H_0 when it is true, and accepting H_1 when it is true. We can also get it wrong by rejecting H_0 when it is really true, and rejecting H_1 when it is really true.

The first of these, rejecting H_0 when it is true, is known as a Type I error. The probability of making this error we initially set at some level, called the level of significance, and this level is conventionally denoted as α. Sometimes, particularly when a computer is used to do the calculations for a test, a p-value may be calculated. This is the probability of finding the observed values, or any values more extreme, given H_0 is true. The complement of significance is called confidence, and in the context of testing statistics is the probability of not rejecting H_0 when it is true.

Rejecting H_0 when H_0 is true is logically equivalent to accepting H_1 when it is false. This can also be known with a probability, conventionally called β. The complement of β $(1 - \beta)$ is known as the *power* of the test, and is the probability of *not* accepting H_0 when it is false, and can be interpreted as the probability of detecting a difference when there is in reality a difference to be detected.

In summary:

- H_0 is a hypothesis of 'no difference'.

- A Type I error is the rejection of H_0 when H_0 is true.

- α is a pre-defined probability, called a significance level, at which making a a Type I error is acceptable.

- A p-value is the probability of finding the observed values, or any values more extreme, given the truth of the null hypothesis.

- Confidence is the complement of significance, that is $1 - \alpha$.

- H_1 is a hypothesis of 'difference'.

- A Type II error is the error of not rejecting H_0 when H_0 is false.

- β is the probability of making a Type II error.

- $1 - \beta$ is called the *power* of a test, and can be interpreted as the probability of detecting a difference if one exists.

Conventionally significance is either set at 5%, or 1%. There is nothing particularly special about these levels; they are arbitrarily selected and not to be taken too seriously. It is for the individual scientist to make up their own minds about whether a particular level of significance is appropriate based on their knowledge of the field of study. Also if a significance is set at 5% it means that *if the null hypothesis were true* we would reject it on 5% of the occasions, that is, make a Type I error. It should not be interpreted as being a probability of the null hypothesis being true or false, and to say so would be an error of interpretation.

Review questions

1. From a sample $n = 10$ of marijuana consignments the THC content has been measured, and the mean found to be 9.5%, the variance being 8.9%.

   (a) What is the probability that the THC content is between 10% and 15%?
   (b) What is the standard error of the mean?
   (c) What is the symmetric 99% confidence interval for the THC in these marijuana consignments?

2. From a sample $n = 10$ of heroin consignments the morphine content has been measured, and the mean found to be 19.38%, the variance being 10.95%.

   (a) What is the 95% confidence interval for the mean?
   (b) What is the 99% confidence interval for the mean?

3. Some brown dog hairs were found on the clothing of a victim of a crime involving a dog. The breadths were measured of five of the hairs and are designated x such that $x = \{46.98, 57.61, 54.25, 51.12, 38.58\}$, and is measured in μm. A suspect has been identified, and is the owner of a dog with similar brown hairs. A sample of five hairs have been taken and their widths measured. These are denoted y, so that $y = \{31.65, 35.30, 50.69, 35.08, 36.60\}$, again the unit of measurement is μm. Is it possible that the hairs found on the victim were left by the suspect's dog?

4. The following table records the observations of the number of cells recovered from water extraction and PBS extraction in an experiment to examine possible differences between the two recovery media with permission from (Martin *et al.*, in press).

Donor	Occasion	No. cells water	No. cells PBS
1	1	1245	1284
1	2	1319	1063
1	3	568	1138
2	1	1675	1666
2	2	1912	3209
2	3	1982	2986
3	1	3103	3209
3	2	1969	1325
3	3	3135	2679

Assume that each occasion for each donor can be considered independent of each other. Is there any evidence for differences between PBS and water recovery?

5 Measures of nominal and ordinal association

The t-test examines significance for differences between observations made on a single variable, but for groupings of observations made from different levels of a factor. In the last section we looked at how Δ^9-THC varied between samples from different years. In a way this is a measure of association between the ordinal variable 'year' and the continuous variable Δ^9-THC, and we were able to tell that, on the basis of the data, the Δ^9-THC concentration in seizures differed between 1986 and 1987. However, what would the strength of that relationship be? We know that there is a 95% confidence that the decrease in concentration is between 0.10% and 1.41%, but what if we had many years' worth of data? Would we see a long-term trend in Δ^9-THC concentration? And, if so, how would we measure the strength of the trend?

This is one of the questions we could answer using some measure of association. In the example above we might wish to know whether there is a significant trend in Δ^9-THC concentration over time. This question could be more directly answered by asking whether there is a significant association between the observations of Δ^9-THC concentration, and the differences in time. This change of inflection may seem to be mere playing about with semantics, but it is at the heart of statistical approaches to data where one tries to link the observable to some explanation of how those observations came to be. The question 'significant trend in time' cannot be answered directly at the level of this book, but the question 'association between time and Δ^9-THC concentration' can be.

Association can be measured for all data types listed in Chapter 2, and for association between different data types. However, measures of association come in so many varieties that this section cannot be exhaustive.

5.1 Association between discrete variables

Often the association sought is between a set of observations measured on a discrete scale, and another set of observations also measured on a discrete scale. These

Introduction to Statistics for Forensic Scientists   David Lucy
© 2005 John Wiley & Sons, Ltd.

observations often take the form of counts, where it is the frequency of observations which constitute the variables.

5.2 χ^2 test for a 2 × 2 table

Perhaps the simplest measure of association is where two variables are nominal and related in some way. Table 5.1 is taken from the work of Katkici *et al.* (1994) and their survey of defence wounds observed during the post-mortem examinations on 195 Turkish victims of all forms of stabbing.

Table 5.1 Observations of defence wounds taken from 195 Turkish victims of all forms of stabbing. Of the 195 victims 162 were male and 33 female. From Katkici *et al.* (1994) reproduced with permission

Sex	Present	Absent	Total
male	57	105	162
female	18	15	33
total	75	120	195

One of the questions in which we may be interested is whether there is any evidence for a difference between the behaviour of males and females during the course of a fatal stabbing. Given the data in Table 5.1 we cannot answer directly whether one sex acts differently during the course of a fatal stabbing attack, but we can look for a significant association between the presence of defence injuries and sex.

From Table 5.1, 57 males and 18 females had defence wounds, so there are more males with defence wounds. However, does this mean that we can infer that males are more likely to defend themselves against a stabbing attack? There are three times as many males with defence wounds, but there are 162 males, and only 33 females in the whole sample, which means there are nearly five times as many males as females in the sample. So does this mean females are more likely to act in such as way as to incur defence wounds?

One statistical test used by statisticians to examine these questions and these data is called the *chi-squared* test. Sometimes the word *chi* is represented by the Greek letter χ, so the test may be denoted as the χ^2-test.

The idea behind the χ^2-test is that for each of k categories there will be an expectation for the count in that category derived from some model. However, the counts actually observed in each of the k categories may differ from those expected counts calculated from the model. Statistical theory shows that as long as each expected value is greater than 1, and that the mean of the expected values exceeds 5, then the variable:

$$\chi^2 = \sum_{i=1}^{k} \frac{(\text{Observed}_i - \text{Expected}_i)^2}{\text{Expected}_i} \qquad (10)$$

is approximated by the χ^2 distribution with $k - 1$ degrees of freedom. This means that, in essence, the probability of observing χ^2, which is a function of the differences between the observed values and the modelled, or expected, values, is distributed χ^2 with $k - 1$ degrees of freedom.

In the example there are four cells, that is k is 4, so $i = \{1, 2, 3, 4\}$, and we have observations of 57 for males and 18 for females with defence injuries, and 105 males and 15 females without defence injuries. But what values would we expect to see?

Following the hypothesis notation in Section 4.5, were the hypothesis (H_0) true, and there were no differences in defence injuries between males and females, then one might expect the numbers of males with and without defence injuries to be the same as the number of females with and without defence injuries relative to the number of males and females in the sample.

We know that the sample comprises a total of 195 individuals, 162 of which are male, and 75 have defence injuries, so we might expect that, of the 75 with defence injuries, 162/195 would be male, so an expected value might be $(75 \times 162)/195 = 62.3$. Similarly, 120 individuals in the sample had no defence injuries, and of those 120 one would expect 162/195 to be male, so an expected number of observations for males without defence injuries is $(120 \times 162)/195 = 99.69$. Likewise, from 195 individuals in the sample there are 33 females, so of the 75 with defence injuries one might expect 33/195 to be female, thus $(75 \times 33)/195 = 12.69$. There is a pattern here, and that is for each cell for which an expected value is to be calculated the corresponding row and column totals are multiplied, then this product is divided by the total sample size. Applying this rule to the final cell, the column total is 120, the row total 33, so the expected value is $(120 \times 33)/195 = 20.31$.

This expected frequencies calculated above only apply when we are assuming that the frequencies should be uniform if all other things are equal. It must be borne in mind that this is not always the case, and that expected values can be drawn from any model one may consider relevant to the question under consideration.

Table 5.1 can be rewritten as below, the expected values being enclosed by parentheses.

Sex	Present	Absent
Male	57 (62.30)	105 (99.69)
female	18 (12.69)	15 (20.31)

From this table observed values and expected values may be substituted into Equation 10. For the cell with the numbers of males with defence injuries the observed value was 57, the expected value is 62.3. The difference between the observed and expected values is −5.3, this squared is 28.09, which is then divided by the expected score of 62.3 to produce the contribution for the cell of 0.45. The contributions from the other cells are calculated in the same way, and are 0.28, 2.22 and 1.39. The sum of these is 4.34.

We now have to turn our attention to the number of degrees of freedom. In the case of cross-classified data the degrees of freedom is given by the number of rows -1 times the number of columns -1. In Table 5.1 there are two rows, and two columns, so the degrees of freedom are $(2 - 1) \times (2 - 1) = 1$.

The final result is that $\chi^2 = 4.34$ with 1 degree of freedom. To calculate a probability for this one may use a function from some statistical software on a computer, however, some critical value may also be looked up in standard statistical tables. If a computer is used then a probability (p-value) of 0.038 is obtained[†], which is the probability of observing the value of χ^2, or any value more extreme given the *null hypothesis*. The null hypothesis in this case is that the expected values are a good model for the observed values. More conventionally one can consult tables such as that in Appendix D. This table is similar to the table of t-distributions in Appendix C in that the tabulation is in the form of three columns, the first column giving the degrees of freedom, and the second column is the value of the parameter χ^2 from Equation 10, where 5% of the probability of that distribution lies beyond the value given in the table. For example, above we calculated χ^2 as 4.34. The value where the 5% tail starts for a χ^2 distribution with one degree of freedom is, by inspection of Appendix D, 3.841. Our calculated value is greater than the tabulated 5% value, thus our calculated value lies well into the 5% region, and would be a value of χ^2 seen less than 5% of the time were the expected values a good model for the observed values. This gives good grounds for rejecting the null hypothesis (H_0) at this level, and acting as though the alternative hypothesis (H_1) were true. The final column in Appendix D is the same as the second column, only these are values for χ^2 at 1% significance. The tabulated value for χ^2 at 1% is 6.635, which is greater than the calculated value of 4.34, so we might expect to see our calculated value more often than 1% of the time were the expected values a good model for the observed values, thus accept (H_0) at the 1% significance level.

The results from our χ^2 test suggest that the differences between the numbers of males with defence wounds, and females with defence wounds in Turkey are significant at the 5% level, but not at the 1% level. This gives us good grounds for believing that there is a real difference between the levels of injuries sustained, but does not from inspection of the table that tell us that much about the strength of the association and, although it is obvious Turkish females have more defence wounds than Turkish males, the test itself gives no indication of the direction of the association between defence wounds and sex.

5.3 Yules *Q*

A useful measure of association for both strength and direction of relationship is Yules Q. Here we think about whether the two properties occur together or not. In the example the two properties would be sex and defence injuries. If we define the

---

[†] On an Excel-like program enter =CHIDIST(4.34,1) into a cell.

property of sex as 'maleness' and males have 'maleness', and females do not have 'maleness', and one has the property of defence injury, or does not have the property of defence injury, then the numbers of those with both properties can be compared with the number of those without both properties and those with one or the other of the properties.

If the 2 × 2 table were to be denoted:

	present	absent
present	A	B
absent	C	D

then a suitable measure of these associations would be:

$$Q = \frac{AD - BC}{AD + BC} \tag{11}$$

where A, B, C and D, are the observed quantities in each cell.

Substituting values from Table 5.1 into Equation 11 we find:

$$Q = \frac{(57 \times 15) - (105 \times 18)}{(57 \times 15) + (105 \times 18)} = -\frac{1035}{2745} = -0.377$$

This means that there is a moderate negative association between defence wounds and 'maleness', which can be restated as a moderate positive association of 0.377 between defence wounds and 'femaleness'.

Yules Q is a very useful measure of association for variables which are in categories, and those categories are exclusive. It can only be used where the table is of a 2 × 2 form. However, extensions to larger tables of exclusive categorical variables are possible and are discussed in some detail in Cohen and Holliday (1982).

Yules Q has the disadvantage that it cannot distinguish a 'complete' association from an 'absolute' association. For instance, a 'complete' association would be one where one of A, B, C, or D takes on the value 0. In this case Q must equal 1 or −1, irrespective of the completeness or otherwise of the other sets of relationships in the table. An 'absolute' relationship is where either A and D or, B and C take the value 0, and is a much stronger relationship. However Yules Q will still equal 1 or −1.

5.4 χ^2 tests for greater than 2 × 2 tables

In the same paper Katkici *et al.* (1994) cross-classify their victims with and without defence wounds by the number of stab wounds. These frequencies are reproduced in Table 5.2.

Here one might expect to see a strong relationship between the presence of defence wounds and the total number of wounds inflicted on the victim as it can be imagined those with only a single stab wound are unlikely to have had a chance to adopt any defensive action. Victims of longer attacks comprising more wounds are more likely to have had an opportunity to defend themselves in some way.

Table 5.2 Observations of defence wounds taken from 195 Turkish victims of stabbing attacks cross classified by the number of wounds. From Katkici *et al.* (1994)

No. wounds	Present	Absent	Total
1	2	58	60
2	3	30	33
3–9	41	22	63
≥ 10	29	10	39
total	75	120	195

Again a χ^2 test is an appropriate starting point. The expected frequencies will be generated from the model that whether a victim has defence wounds or not is unrelated to the number of wounds they have received.

As before, the expected frequencies under the model for each cell are calculated by multiplying the appropriate column and row totals and dividing by the total number in the sample, so for the top left-hand cell in Table 5.2 the expected frequency is $(60 \times 75)/195 = 23.08$. The observed and expected frequencies are listed here, the expected frequencies in parentheses:

	Present	Absent
1	2 (23.08)	58 (36.92)
2	3 (12.69)	30 (20.30)
3–9	41 (24.23)	22 (38.77)
≥ 10	29 (15.00)	10 (24.00)

Substituting these values into Equation 10 the variable $X^2 = 19.25 + 7.40 + 11.61 + 13.07 + 12.03 + 4.63 + 7.25 + 8.17 = 83.41$. As there are four rows and two columns then there are 3 df. Inspection of Appendix D gives $\chi^2 = 7.81$ at 5%, and $\chi^2 = 11.34$ at 1% with 3 df. The calculated value of χ^2 is 83.41, which is a more extreme value than either of the tabulated values. This means that the differences are significant at a level greater than 1%, and we have good justification to act as though the alternative hypothesis (H_1) were true.

But what is the strength of the relationship between the presence and absence of defence wounds and the number of wounds?

5.5 ϕ^2 and Cramers V^2

Despite the differences calculated above being highly significant this does not necessarily mean that the presence and absence of defence wounds is highly related to the number of wounds seen on victims of fatal stabbings. One of the properties of the χ^2 test is that variables showing only a weak relationship can exhibit highly significant values of χ^2; this is because if we inspect Equation 10, the value of χ^2 is proportional to counts. So, were one to have a cell where the observed value is 20, and the expected value 10, then the contribution to χ^2 would be 10. Contrast this with a cell where the observed value was 40, and the expected value 20. This cell would contribute a value of 20 to χ^2. The relationship between the observed and expected values has been maintained, but the contribution to χ^2 has increased simply by increasing the sample size. This might make sense in terms of being more confident about the existence of a relationship because we are basing our knowledge of the existence on a greater number of observations, but it tells us little about the actual strength of the relationship. One of the drawbacks of the χ^2 test is that, if an association between two variables exists, no matter how small that relationship, highly significant results can be obtained simply by increasing the sample size.

One way in which the value of χ^2 can be changed to account for the sample size is simply to divide it by the sample size. This measure is known as $\phi^{2\ddagger}$, and has the convenient property for a 2×2 table, or table where there are either two rows or two columns, of taking the value zero for no relationship, and the value one for a perfect relationship. For the example above the value of χ^2 was 83.41, and the sample size 195, so $\phi^2 = 83.41/195 = 0.45$, which we know from the testing above to be a significant relationship, but because the value is closer to zero than one is quite a weak one.

ϕ^2 is useful for $2 \times k$ tables, where either the number of rows or the number of columns is equal to two, but is not so useful for $n \times k$ tables, where it is possible for ϕ^2 to be greater than 1. In these cases ϕ^2 may itself be standardized. The best known of these standardizations is Cramers V^2, where:

$$V^2 = \frac{\phi^2}{\min(n-1, k-1)}$$

where n may be the number of rows and k the number of columns.

5.6 The limitations of χ^2 testing

There are a number of points to be borne in mind when considering the χ^2 test. These are:

1. It is easy to take statistical significance more seriously than it warrants. With significance testing of all types statistically significant results should be used more as a springboard from which to make further conjectures about the substantive nature of the matter in hand, and if possible be accompanied by further testing on

---

$\ddagger$ Pronounced phi squared, where *ph* is pronounced *f*.

the strength of relationships. They should not be treated as any sort of definitive answer in their own right.

2. In the particular case of the χ^2 test every expected frequency should be greater than 1, and their mean should be greater then 5. If the first criterion is not met, and the data ordinal, then it is possible to amalgamate categories until the frequencies in each cell are sufficient. If the mean of the expected values is below 5 then more data are needed.

3. The χ^2 test can only be used to look for deviations from a model for *count* data. It should not be used for proposition data such as percentages.

What of the defence wounds?

Earlier in this section the question was posed whether males and females in Turkey acted differently during the course of a fatal stabbing. There are certainly differences between the numbers of females and males who showed defence wounds, and who subsequently died, but just what this means is open to interpretation. The strength of the relationship is 0.377, which is a modest relationship, but it is statistically significant at a level smaller than 5%. It could be that Turkish women who are attacked are more likely to try to defend themselves than their male counterparts, or that there are systematic and unseen differences in the nature of the attacks. One point is that all these victims died as a result of the attack. Possibly males who resist are more likely to resist in a way which deters the attack so they do not die, whereas women who resist might be less effective in that resistance. On the other hand the deaths observed by Katkici *et al.* (1994) are from all stabbing deaths. Could it not be that males are more likely to commit suicide with a bladed weapon?

Katkici *et al.* (1994) went on to examine defence wounds with the age of the victim, blood alcohol levels, and the exact area upon which the defence injuries occurred. They concluded that absence of defence injury does not ignore that an attack did not take place, but presence of defence injury could be used as a strong indication that an attack did take place. It is evident that, whatever the true explanation for male/female defence wound differences, it is for the forensic scientist to infer explanations from data. Statistical testing is likely to be of assistance in this process, but the fundamental inferential method rests with the imagination and experience of the scientist.

5.7 Interpretation and conclusions

The statistical interpretation of tests such as the χ^2 test is the same as for the t-test, and is outlined in Section 4.7. It does not mean that there is a 95% probability of association if the null hypothesis is rejected, nor is there a 95% probability that there is no association if it is not rejected. The significance probability simply refers to the probability of making a Type I error.

Even if it is accepted that there is a strong association between two variables, there is no necessary causal connection between the two. The statistical association may just be a coincidence of observation, or the association may caused by a third unobserved variable to which both are causally linked, but the two have no direct causal effect upon each other. A method for investigating this type of interrelationship will be explored in Section 6.4. Unexpected strong associations should be treated with a little scepticism unless causal explanations can be sought from background theory.

Review questions

1. In their work on serial sexual homicide in Virginia (USA) McNamara and Morton (2004, Table 2, reproduced with permission) give the following table of numbers of murders per year.

Year	Murders
1987	437
1988	468
1989	480
1990	545
1991	584
1992	563
1993	539
1994	570
1995	501
1996	496

Is there any evidence to support the notion that the number of murders are related to year?

2. Pittella and Gusmao (2003) observed diffuse vascular injuries (DVI), and diffuse axonal injuries (DAI) in the brains of 120 road accident fatalities. From 120 victims they found the following (Pittella and Gusmao, 2003, Table 2, reproduced with permission):

DVI	DAI	
	present	absent
present	14	0
absent	82	24

What is the strength of relationship between DVI and DAI in these victims?

3. De Kinder (2002) investigated the effects of the use of a firearm upon the consistency of rifling marks made upon the projectile and the breech face of a cartridge. For this study De Kinder used many of the types of firearm in a test project seen in casework. The table (reproduced with permission) below is a sub-set of the table given by De Kinder and shows the numbers of each type of firearm.

Firearm	Project	Casework
0.177 air	3	12
0.22	68	23
6.35 Browning	8	14
7.65 Browning	11	41
9mm parabellum	17	32

Are the types of firearm used by De Kinder in the project any different from those encountered in casework?

4. Gülekon and Turgut (2003) examined three types of external occipital protuberance (EOP) in relation to the sex of an individual. The three types were: type I – a less prominent bump, type II – a crest, and, type III – a spine. They made a radiological examination of 500 women, and 500 men from an Anatolian population. The table below is a cross-tabulation of EOP by sex, and is taken from Table 1 of Gülekon and Turgut (2003, reproduced with permission):

Type	Women	Men
type I	427	89
type II	52	94
type III	21	317

Is there a significant relationship between EOP and sex, and what is the strength of this relationship?

6

Correlation

In the last few sections we have examined whether there is a relationship between variables, and some methods for measuring the strengths of those relationships for when the data is of a count form. However, many variables, particularly those measured in the laboratory, tend to be on a continuous scale. Examples would be elemental concentrations, time, and most machine responses.

The term statisticians use for the measurement of strength of relationship between continuous variables is correlation. Any continuous variables which have some sort of systematic relationship are said to covary, and any variable which covaries with any other is said to be a covariate. This terminology can be used for any discrete variables as well as those which are continuous in nature, but the terms are more commonly used in the continuous case.

A basic tool for the investigation of correlation is the *scatterplot*. Usually only two variables are plotted, but three can be accommodated. Scatterplots with representations any more than three axes are difficult to interpret.

A statistical measure of correlation is called the correlation coefficient. This is calculated in such a way that it can only take on values between -1 and 1. A value of correlation coefficient of 1 means that the variables are absolutely related, as does a value of -1. A value -1 means that the two variables are absolutely related, but that as one increases, the other decreases. A value of zero means that the variables are unrelated.

Correlation can be thought of as a strength of relationship. The strength of relationship is independent of the form of relationship. Most commonly linear relationships are considered, where the relationship between covariates can be thought of as a straight line. It is, however, possible in other forms of relationship. After linear relationships log relationships of some form are the most common, although for the moment we shall consider relationships between variables which are linear in form. Figure 6.1 gives bivariate scatterplots of varying linear correlation coefficients.

Introduction to Statistics for Forensic Scientists   David Lucy
© 2005 John Wiley & Sons, Ltd.

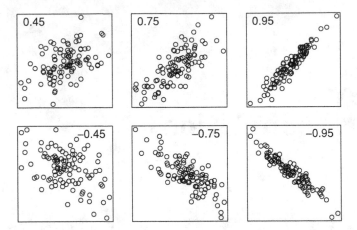

Figure 6.1 Scatterplots for six sets of bivariate data of varying linear correlation coefficients. The top row have correlation coefficients which are positive, where increase in one of the variables is followed by an increase in the other. The bottom row have negative correlation coefficients, which means that an increase in one of the variables is followed by a decrease in the other

The graphs in Figure 6.1 show bivariate datasets which have a positive linear correlation on the top row, and a negative linear correlation on the bottom row. The magnitudes of the correlation coefficients are arranged so that the least highly correlated is on the left, the most highly correlated being on the right. The higher the correlation, that is the further the correlation coefficient is from zero, the more the scatter of points resembles a single line of points. The low correlations of 0.45 at the left-hand side of Figure 6.1 resemble more closely a random scatter of points in the area of the graph, and were the correlation coefficient zero they would be a random scatter.

To demonstrate the process involved in the calculation of a linear correlation coefficient an example will be used. Grim *et al.* (2002) used laser desorption mass spectrometry to examine the ageing properties of the dye methyl violet, a common dye used in inks from the 1950s. Using a series of controlled experiments on various inks containing methyl violet Grim *et al.* (2002) artificially aged documents with ultra violet (UV) radiation. After various times the average molecular weight for the methyl violet compound was measured. The observations from one of these experiments on a 1950s document are given in Table 6.1.

The first thing to do is to plot the data from Table 6.1 to see what they look like, and to gain some feel for these particular data. Figure 6.2 gives irradiation time on the *x* axis and average molecular weight on the *y* axis. Visual inspection of Figure 6.2 would suggest that there is a negative linear correlation between these two variables.

What we should like to know is 'what is the strength of this relationship?'. The trend of the points in Figure 6.2 look linear, and is in one direction only, that is, the relationship is monotonic. A suitable measure of this linear correlation r is

Table 6.1 Average molecular weight of the dye methyl violet and UV irradiation time from an accelerated ageing experiment. From Grim *et al.* (2002, Figure 9)

Time (min)	Weight (Da)
0.0	367.20
15.3	368.97
30.6	367.42
45.3	366.19
60.2	365.91
75.5	365.68
90.6	365.12
105.7	363.59

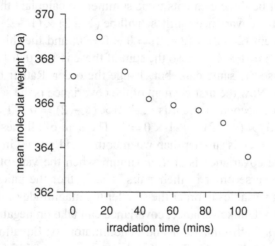

Figure 6.2 Scatterplot of x UV irradiation time and y average molecular weight of methyl violet ions. There is a marked negative linear correlation between these two covariates

given by:

$$r = \frac{\sum(x_i - \bar{x})(y_i - \bar{y})}{\sqrt{\{\sum(x_i - \bar{x})^2 \sum(y_i - \bar{y})^2\}}} \tag{12}$$

The two terms in the denominator of Equation 12 we have come across before. In Section 2.5 in page 13 the variance was given as:

$$\text{variance} = \frac{\sum(x_i - \bar{x})}{(n-1)}$$

The two terms in the denominator are simply the numerator of the variance of the two sets of observations. For the x variable, which is irradiation time, the mean is 52.89, and for the y variable, average molecular weight, the mean is 366.26.

The numerator from Equation 12 looks similar to the term for variance, but is termed the covariance. Covariances on their own do not really mean very much, but in statistical science are one of the most important quantities as they are used in many other more advanced statistical methods. Put simply, the covariance is a measure of the extent to which small values in one variable are paired with small values in the other variable, and how large variables in one are paired with large values in the other. This can, of course, be the other way around, that is, small values with large ones and large values with small ones, but the essential point is that it is a measure of how the pairs are ordered.

Take for instance two variables x and y and we shall make both of these $x = y = \{1, 2, 3\}$. The mean of both x and y is 2. As there are three pairs of points in x and y, there will be three elements to be summed to calculate the covariance. The first element of the covariance for these will be $(1 - 2) \times (1 - 2) = -1 \times -1 = 1$, the second element $(2 - 2) \times (2 - 2) = 0 \times 0 = 0$, and the third element will be $(3 - 2) \times (3 - 2) = 1 \times 1 = 1$. So the sum of these is $1 + 0 + 1 = 2$.

Let us now use the same data, but change the order. Rather than $y = \{1, 2, 3\}$, let $y = \{1, 3, 2\}$. Now the first element of the covariance is the same as before, that is 1, however, the second element is $(2 - 2) \times (3 - 2) = 0 \times 1 = 0$, and the third element is $(2 - 3) \times (2 - 2) = -1 \times 0 = 0$. The sum of all these elements is now $1 + 0 + 0 = 1$, which is smaller than when both x and y were in the same order.

In general the covariance is at a maximum when the variables are in order in their pairs, or reverse order in their pairs. The further the pairs are from having their constituent variables in order the smaller the magnitude of the covariance to a minimum of zero. Unlike variance, covariance can take on negative values.

The values for both numerator and denominator for Equation 12 for the data from Table 6.1 are tabulated in Table 6.2. $\sum\{(x - \bar{x})^2\} = 9545.50$, $\sum\{(y - \bar{y})^2\} =$

Table 6.2 Table of values for $x - \bar{x}$, $(x - \bar{x})^2$, $y - \bar{y}$, $(y - \bar{x})^2$ and $(x - \bar{x})(x - \bar{x})$ for the calculation of the linear correlation coefficient between average molecular weight and UV irradiation time for the data from Table 6.1.

Time (min)	$x - \bar{x}$	$(x - \bar{x})^2$	Weight (Da)	$y - \bar{y}$	$(y - \bar{y})^2$	$(x - \bar{x})(y - \bar{y})$
0.0	−52.90	2798.41	367.20	0.94	0.883	−49.72
15.3	−37.61	1414.51	368.97	2.71	7.344	−101.92
30.6	−22.33	498.63	367.42	1.16	1.345	−25.90
45.3	−7.61	57.91	366.19	−0.07	0.005	0.53
60.2	7.33	53.73	365.91	−0.35	0.122	−2.57
75.5	22.61	511.21	365.68	−0.58	0.336	−13.11
90.6	37.67	1419.03	365.12	−1.14	1.300	−42.94
105.7	52.84	2792.06	363.59	−2.67	7.129	−141.08
$\bar{x} = 52.89$		$\sum 545.50$	$\bar{y} = 366.26$		$\sum 18.465$	$\sum -376.72$

18.465, and the covariance between x and y is $(x - \bar{x})(y - \bar{y}) = -376.72$. Substituting these values into Equation 12 we have:

$$r = \frac{-376.72}{\sqrt{9545.50 \times 18.465}} = \frac{-376.72}{419.83} = -0.8973$$

The linear correlation coefficient between the average molecular weight for methyl violet ions and the UV irradiation time is ≈ -0.89. This means that as the irradiation time increases the average molecular weight of methyl violet ions decreases, and, as 0.89 quite close to -1, the negative linear relationship is quite strong.

6.1 Significance tests for correlation coefficients

Above we found that the linear correlation coefficient between average molecular weight of methyl violet ions and UV irradiation time was -0.89. This value sounds quite high, but is it significantly high? Is it not possible that such a linear correlation coefficient would occur from data drawn randomly from a bivariate normal distribution with zero covariance?

Also, how about the effect of the sample size? It makes sense that a high linear correlation coefficient based on lots of xy pairs is somehow more significant than an equal linear correlation coefficient based on only a few observations, and some sort of evaluation of the significance of the linear correlation coefficient may be appropriate.

It turns out that, for the hypothesis that the correlation coefficient r is zero, a suitable test statistic is (Myres, 1990):

$$t = \frac{r \times \sqrt{df}}{\sqrt{1 - r^2}} \tag{13}$$

where the value t is an ordinate on the t-distribution with df refers to degrees of freedom. In the case of methyl violet ions and UV irradiation time the linear correlation coefficient was -0.89 and this was based on 8 xy pairs. The degrees of freedom are equal to $n - 2$ where there are n xy pairs, so in this case there are 6 df. Substituting 6 for df and -0.89 for r into 13 we have:

$$t = \frac{-0.89 \times \sqrt{6}}{\sqrt{1 - -0.89^2}} = -4.78$$

This is an ordinate on the t-distribution with 6 df. Appendix C has values for the 95th and 99th percentile of t-distributions with various degrees of freedom. If we look at Appendix C for the values of a t-distribution with degrees of freedom equal to 6 we see that 95% of the area is within ± 2.447. Our value of -4.78 is an ordinate beyond -2.447, so we can say that the linear correlation coefficient is significant at 95% confidence. The value of the ordinate t at 99% is 3.707. Again the value of -4.78 which is the ordinate calculated from Equation 13 is greater in magnitude than the tabulated value, so it is a value more extreme than 99% of the distribution, thus the value of -4.78 is significant at the 99% level of confidence.

6.2 Correlation coefficients for non-linear data

Andrasko and Ståhling (1998) measured three compounds associated with the discharge of firearms, naphthalene, TEAC-2 and nitroglycerin, over a period of time by solid phase microextraction (SPME) of the gaseous residue from the expended cartridge. They found that the concentrations of these three compounds would decrease with time, and that this property would be of use in estimating the time since discharge for these types of cartridges.

Table 6.3 is a table of the peak area for nitroglycerine and time elapsed since discharge for a Winchester SKEET 100 cartridge stored at 7°C. These data are represented as a series of three scatterplots in Figure 6.3.

Table 6.3 Table of values for time since discharge in days of a shotgun cartridge and height of a peak associated with nitroglycerin. The cartridge was stored at 7°C. From Andrasko and Ståhling (1998, Figure 3)

Time since discharge (days)	Nitroglycerin (peak height)
1.21	218.34
2.42	216.16
3.62	100.00
4.69	75.55
7.49	56.52
9.42	50.62
11.60	31.00
14.69	41.44
21.50	15.53
25.70	14.63
29.86	10.41
37.20	5.16
42.42	7.26

Figure 6.3(a) shows a scattergram where the covariates, peak height of nitroglycerin and time since discharge are fairly evidently not linearly related. The fall in the peak height associated with nitroglycerin is much greater with time than would be expected were the fall to be linear. Despite the self-evident non-linearity the linear correlation coefficient is −0.73, which is quite high.

The high linear correlation (−0.73) for data which is obviously not linear in relationship does not truly represent the strength of the relationship. That is, the true strength of relationship is lost because we are simply imposing the wrong model upon the data. So what can we do about it?

A linear relationship is not an unreasonable starting assumption, in that we know nitroglycerin will be lost with time, however, we now know this loss is not linear.

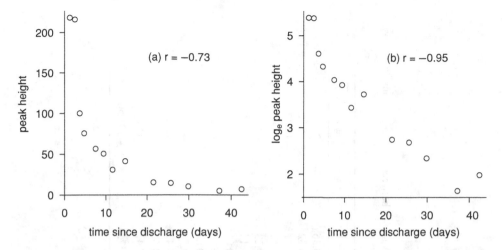

Figure 6.3 Two scatterplots of the peak height of nitroglycerin sampled from the barrel of a shotgun (Winchester – cartridge SKEET 100) and the time in days since the last discharge of that firearm. (a) is the data from Table 6.3 unaltered, (b) is a $\log_{10}$(Peak height) against linear time scatterplot. The linear correlation coefficients are in the top left-hand corner of each scatterplot

A common model for loss in chemistry is called an exponential decay model, and entails a log-linear relationship between the two variables. The centre scatterplot of Figure 6.3 shows the $\log_e{}^\dagger$ of the nitroglycerine peak height against linear time. Here we can see that the relationship looks very much more linear. In fact the linear correlation coefficient is -0.95, which is high, and suggests that this may be a realistic transformation of the variables. The calculations for the log-linear correlation coefficient are exactly the same kind as in Table 6.2, only the $\log_e$ of the y variable has been used, rather than the untransformed y. To clear any confusion these are tabulated in Table 6.4.

Substituting values from Table 6.4 into Equation 12 we have:

$$r = \frac{-191.56}{\sqrt{2203.90 \times 17.80}} = -0.95$$

which is a considerable increase in linear correlation coefficient over the -0.73 produced from the untransformed values for the nitroglycerin peak height, and suggests that the true relationship is of a log-linear form.

Andrasko and Ståhling (1998) measured several different types of discharged cartridge stored under several different temperature regimens. Their findings suggested that measurements of naphthalene and TEAC-2 compounds were the most suitable if time since discharge estimation is the object of the measurement process. They also found some variation within batches of the same cartridge type provided by the same manufacturer.

$\dagger$ Andrasko and Ståhling (1998) used $\log_{10}$ of the nitroglycerin peak against linear time. Conventionally $\log_e$ would be used, although mathematically it makes no difference.

Table 6.4 Table of values for x, $x - \bar{x}$, $(x - \bar{x})^2$, y, $\log y$ and $(\log x - \overline{\log y})$, and the covariance between x and $\log y$ from the data in Table 6.3.

x	$x - \bar{x}$	$(x - \bar{x})^2$	y	$\log y$	$\log y - \overline{\log y}$	$(\log y - \overline{\log y})^2$	$(x - \bar{x})(\log y - \overline{\log y})$
1.21	−15.08	227.52	218.34	5.39	1.83	3.36	−27.64
2.42	−13.87	192.48	216.16	5.38	1.82	3.32	−25.28
3.62	−12.67	160.63	100	4.61	1.05	1.11	−13.32
4.69	−11.6	134.65	75.55	4.32	0.77	0.59	−8.94
7.49	−8.8	77.51	56.52	4.03	0.48	0.23	−4.23
9.42	−6.87	47.25	50.62	3.92	0.37	0.14	−2.55
11.6	−4.69	22.03	31	3.43	−0.12	0.01	0.56
14.69	−1.6	2.57	41.44	3.72	0.17	0.03	−0.27
21.5	5.21	27.1	15.53	2.74	−0.81	0.66	−4.22
25.7	9.41	88.48	14.63	2.68	−0.87	0.76	−8.19
29.86	13.57	184.04	10.41	2.34	−1.21	1.47	−16.43
37.2	20.91	437.07	5.16	1.64	−1.91	3.66	−39.99
42.42	26.13	682.58	7.26	1.98	−1.57	2.47	−41.06
$\bar{x} = 16.29$		$\sum 2203.90$		$\overline{\log y} = 3.55$		$\sum 17.80$	$\sum −191.56$

6.3 The coefficient of determination

A quantity often associated with the correlation coefficient is the *coefficient of determination,* which is a direct measure of how much of the variance in one of the covariates is attributed to the other. Imagine on Figure 6.3(b) that there is a line which goes through the scatter of points describing the relationship between the two covariates. We can imagine that the total variance in nitroglycerin peak height is made up of two parts, that which is attributable to the relationship with x (time), and that which can be seen as random noise about the line. The coefficient of determination is a quantity describing what proportion of the variance is attributable to the relationship described by the line.

The coefficient of determination is easy to calculate, it is simply the square of the correlation coefficient. For instance, in the log transformed data above the correlation coefficient was -0.95, which means that the coefficient of determination is $-0.95^2 = 0.90$. Often the coefficient of determination is described as a percentage, which, in the example above, means that 90% of the variance in nitroglycerin peak area is attributable to time.

Sometimes the coefficient of determination when cited as a percentage is known as the 'percentage level of variation', and is considered a more realistic measure of the strength of a linear relationship than the correlation coefficient.

6.4 Partial correlation

A high correlation or statistical level of association may lead to the conclusion that there is some basis for the association, indeed that one may cause in some material sense the other, however, unobserved causal links cannot legitimately be inferred simply by association between covariates. That is, there is no logically compelling reason to accept that there is a causal link between covariates simply on the basis of association no matter how reasonable it might be to suppose that there is.

This is one of the problems with statistical association, and in fact all sciences of which learning by experience, or induction, is a part. The fact that universal rules have to be inferred from observations which are not themselves open to direct experience leaves something of a logical gap in scientific methodology.

So what can go wrong? Mostly, philosophical considerations aside, it would be foolish to treat covariates exhibiting high correlations as being unrelated unless there were some very good reason for believing so. But also we have to ask whether we really care about whether there is an underlying causal effect between covariates or not. In forensic science we are trying to make inferences about problems such as matching and past activities. Does it really matter, for example, that we have no logical reason to infer the presence of a causal mechanism which explains the decrease in nitroglycerin peak height with time? If our purpose is to make inferences about the time since discharge of a cartridge causation, although pleasant, it is not absolutely necessary to know that there is a causal mechanism so long as the relationship between time since discharge and nitroglycerin peak height remains a constant. Of course, were we to be able to infer a necessary causal relationship then we would be able to guarantee that the relationship would always be there. The fact that the relationship does not exist in any guaranteed sense does little to deter us from using the fact that there seems to be a constant conjunction between nitroglycerin peak height and time since discharge to make estimates for time since discharge for cartridges for which we have not directly observed.

Another problem, and one for which statistical science has a form of answer, is that a relationship may not exist directly between two observable covariates, but that the appearance of direct causation is merely an impression given by the fact that both the covariates are in themselves covariates of a hidden variable. That is, there may be no direct relationship between nitroglycerin peak height and time, but that both are independent of each other, but dependent on some third, unseen, covariate. This would result in an extreme case of independence being masked by a third variable. A more common set of relationships would be when the covariates are all linked to each other in some way.

Gerostamoulos and Drummer (2000) recorded the concentrations of morphine and metabolites in blood from 21 cases where death had been caused by heroin taking. They recorded the concentrations of morphine-3-glucuronide, morphine-6-glucuronide and free morphine in the femoral region of the cadaver immediately after admission to the mortuary, and at the time of post mortem. Their data is recorded in Table 6.5. A sub-set for morphine-3-glucuronide on admission, morphine-6-glucuronide on admission, and free morphine measured during the post-mortem examination is repeated in Table 6.6.

For this example we shall not calculate the individual correlation coefficients by hand, as we did above 4.6, but calculate them by computer. The correlation coefficients for the variables in Table 6.6 are given in Table 6.7. Table 6.7 is, for clarity, an upper triangle of the full correlation table. The dashes do not indicate that there is no value in those positions, but rather that, for example, the correlation between morphine-3-glucuronide during post-mortem examination (M3 post mortem) and morphine-3-glucuronide upon admission (M3 admission) is 0.818, therefore the correlation between morphine-3-glucuronide upon admission (M3 admission) and morphine-3-glucuronide during post-mortem examination (M3 post mortem) will also be 0.818, as correlation gives no sense of the direction of relationship, so there is no need to put the value in the table as the upper triangle gives all the necessary values and is easier to read than the full table. It should also be noticed that the leading diagonal of Table 6.7 consists of 1's. The reason for this is that these are the correlation coefficients for each variable with itself, which is bound to be 1. Again these could be dispensed with entirely, but the table is clearer to read with them left in.

As morphine-3-glucuronide is a metabolite of free morphine one can expect the quantities of morphine-3-glucuronide to depend on the quantities of free morphine,

Table 6.5 Concentrations of morphine and metabolites in post-mortem and admission blood from 20 cases. M3G – morphine-3-glucuronide, M6G – morphine-6-glucuronide, FM – free morphine, TM – total morphine. Reproduced with Gerostamoulos and Drummer (2000, Table 2); case 15 has been omitted because of incomplete data

Case	M3G admission	M3G post mortem	M6G admission	M6G post mortem	FM admission	FM post mortem
1	0.55	0.63	0.09	0.1	0.18	0.23
2	0.22	0.07	0.05	0.09	0.21	0.17
3	0.69	0.58	0.21	0.08	0.14	0.13
4	1.6	1.2	0.3	0.12	0.8	0.8
5	0.75	0.39	0.16	0.99	0.4	0.15
6	2.2	2.5	0.5	0.45	0.27	0.27
7	1.7	2.1	0.32	0.39	0.26	0.45
8	0.36	0.66	0.08	0.22	0.08	0.07
9	0.16	1.4	0.02	0.11	0.71	0.36
10	0.3	0.17	0.06	0.12	0.7	1.2
11	0.27	0.15	0.07	0.05	0.2	0.08
12	0.55	0.9	0.16	0.15	0.21	0.19
13	1.2	0.78	0.38	0.17	0.69	0.9
14	0.57	0.31	0.17	0.27	0.08	0.19
16	0.78	1.1	0.23	0.58	0.36	1.92
17	0.2	0.27	0.02	0.02	0.5	0.41
18	0.32	0.26	0.18	0.06	0.08	0.05
19	0.15	0.15	0.1	0.05	0.36	0.16
20	0.63	0.45	0.08	0.09	0.21	0.5
21	0.5	0.56	0.09	0.1	0.17	0.12

but not the other way round. We would not expect the quantities of free morphine during post-mortem examination to depend on the quantities of morphine-3-glucuronide either on admission, or on post-mortem examination, however, the quantities of morphine-3-glucuronide during post-mortem examination may depend on the quantities of free morphine during post-mortem examination. Similarly, we might expect the quantities of morphine-3-glucuronide during the post-mortem examination to depend on the quantities of morphine-3-glucuronide during admission, but not the other way round. In fact the quantities of free morphine during post-mortem examination should not depend on the quantities of any of its metabolites.

So why is it that the quantities of free morphine during admission are unexpectedly correlated, albeit at a fairly low level (0.206), with morphine-3-glucuronide measured during admission? The answer is that both are related indirectly through morphine-3-glucuronide measured during the post-mortem examination.

One quantity in which we may be interested is the correlation coefficient between morphine-3-glucuronide measured upon admission with free morphine during the post-mortem examination were they not mutually linked via morphine-3-glucuronide

Table 6.6 Morphine concentrations taken from femoral blood from 20 cases. In their original work Gerostamoulos and Drummer (2000, Table 6.2) examined 21 cases, but case 15 has been omitted here because complete data was not available for it. M3G – morphine-3-glucuronide, FM – free morphine. These were measured both on admission and at post mortem, a fuller table of Gerostamoulos and Drummer's data is given in Table 6.5

Case	M3 admission	M3 post mortem	FM post mortem
1	0.55	0.63	0.23
2	0.22	0.07	0.17
3	0.69	0.58	0.13
4	1.60	1.20	0.80
5	0.75	0.39	0.15
6	2.20	2.50	0.27
7	1.70	2.10	0.45
8	0.36	0.66	0.07
9	0.16	1.20	0.36
10	0.30	0.17	1.20
11	0.27	0.15	0.08
12	0.55	0.90	0.19
13	1.20	0.78	0.90
14	0.57	0.31	0.19
16	0.78	1.10	1.92
17	0.20	0.27	0.41
18	0.32	0.26	0.05
19	0.15	0.15	0.16
20	0.63	0.45	0.50
21	0.50	0.56	0.12

Table 6.7 The upper triangle of the correlation table for morphine concentrations taken from femoral blood from 20 cadavers. The featured covariates are morphine-3-glucuronide upon admission (M3 admission), morphine-3-glucuronide during post-mortem examination (M3 post mortem), and free morphine during post-mortem examination (FM post mortem)

	M3 admission	M3 post mortem	FM post mortem
M3 admission	1.000	0.818	0.206
M3 post mortem	–	1.000	0.174
FM post mortem	–	–	1.000

measured at post-mortem examination. The quantity in which we might be interested is called the partial correlation coefficient between morphine-3-glucuronide on admission and free morphine during post-mortem examination.

Partial correlation coefficients are very similar to the linear correlation coefficients we have been dealing with up to now except they take into account correlations with other variables in the data. But first we need some terminology.

Let us denote morphine-3-glucuronide measured upon admission as 1, morphine-3-glucuronide measured at post-mortem examination as 2, free morphine measured during the post-mortem examination as 3, and any correlation coefficient as r. It is then possible to refer to the correlation coefficient between morphine-3-glucuronide measured upon admission and morphine-3-glucuronide measured at post-mortem examination as r_{12}, where the subscripts refer to the variables. So referring to Table 6.7, $r_{12} = 0.818$, $r_{13} = 0.206$, and $r_{23} = 0.174$. Obviously $r_{12} = r_{21} = 0.82$ and so on.

Now let $r_{12|3}$ mean the correlation coefficient of morphine-3-glucuronide measured upon admission with morphine-3-glucuronide measured at post-mortem examination *given* free morphine measured during the post-mortem examination. The vertical line means *given*, and in this context means controlling for the effects of free morphine measured during the post-mortem examination.

In the specific case for these three variables:

$$r_{12|3} = \frac{r_{12} - r_{13}\, r_{23}}{\sqrt{1 - r_{13}^2}\sqrt{1 - r_{23}^2}}$$

So:

$$r_{12|3} = \frac{0.818 - (0.206 \times 0.174)}{\sqrt{1 - 0.206^2}\sqrt{1 - 0.174^2}} = \frac{0.782}{0.978 \times 0.985} = 0.811,$$

0.811 being the partial correlation coefficient between morphine-3-glucuronide measured upon admission and morphine-3-glucuronide measured at post-mortem examination controlling for free morphine measured during the post-mortem examination. As can be seen this is not very different from the value of 0.818 obtained when the free morphine is not controlled for.

A more general expression for a partial correlation coefficient between two variables, call them i and j, given a third variable k is:

$$r_{ij|k} = \frac{r_{ij} - r_{ik}\, r_{jk}}{\sqrt{1 - r_{ik}^2}\sqrt{1 - r_{jk}^2}} \tag{14}$$

So, to calculate the partial correlation coefficient between morphine-3-glucuronide measured upon admission and free morphine measured during the post-mortem examination controlling for the effects of morphine-3-glucuronide measured at post-mortem examination, we can substitute morphine-3-glucuronide measured upon admission for i, free morphine measured during the post-mortem examination for j and morphine-3-glucuronide measured at post-mortem examination for k, this gives:

$$r_{13|2} = \frac{0.206 - (0.818 \times 0.174)}{\sqrt{1 - 0.818^2}\sqrt{1 - 0.174^2}} = \frac{0.064}{0.575 \times 0.985} = 0.113$$

For the partial correlation between morphine-3-glucuronide measured at post-mortem examination and free morphine measured during the post-mortem examination given morphine-3-glucuronide measured upon admission.

$$r_{23|1} = \frac{0.174 - (0.818 \times 0.206)}{\sqrt{1 - 0.818^2}\sqrt{1 - 0.206^2}} = \frac{0.006}{0.575 \times 0.979} = 0.011$$

The three partial correlation coefficients can be arranged in a table similar to Table 6.7 and are given in Table 6.8.

Table 6.8 Partial correlation table for the variables featured in Table 6.7. The variable notation is unchanged

	M3 admission	M3 post mortem	FM post mortem
M3 admission	1.000	0.811	0.113
M3 post mortem	–	1.000	0.011
FM post mortem	–	–	1.000

The only respect in which the partial correlations for these three covariates are changed from the correlation coefficients is that the relationship with free morphine and the two metabolites has been reduced. The partial correlation of morphine-3-glucuronide measured upon admission and free morphine measured during the post-mortem examination has been reduced to 0.113, and between morphine-3-glucuronide measured during post-mortem examination and free morphine measured during the post-mortem examination has been reduced to 0.011.

Testing a partial correlation coefficient is exactly the same as testing a non-partialed correlation coefficient, except the degrees of freedom are calculated in a slightly different way. A test statistic for partial correlations is given by Equation 13 in Section 6.1, but in the case of a partial correlation coefficient the degrees of freedom are calculated from the number of rows in the data minus the number of variables. From Table 6.6 there are 20 rows and three variables, so there are 17 df.

The value t is an ordinate on in the relevant t-distribution defined by the degrees of freedom. These are already tabulated in Appendix D. So for 17 df a critical value at 95% confidence for t is 2.11. A value of t for the partial correlation between morphine-3-glucuronide measured upon admission and morphine-3-glucuronide measured during post-mortem examination is:

$$t = \frac{0.814 \times \sqrt{17}}{\sqrt{1 - 0.814^2}} = \frac{3.35}{0.581} = 5.78,$$

which is larger than the tabulated critical value of 2.11, therefore the partial correlation is significant at the 95% level. For the partial correlation of 0.113 between morphine-3-glucuronide measured upon admission and free morphine at the post-mortem examination the value of the test statistic t is:

$$t = \frac{0.113 \times \sqrt{17}}{\sqrt{1 - 0.113^2}} = \frac{0.466}{0.993} = 0.469,$$

which is less than the critical value of the test statistic, so this partial correlation is not significant at a 95% confidence level. The final partial correlation between morphine-3-glucuronide measured at the post-mortem examination and free morphine at the post-mortem examination is much smaller than the previous partial correlation which is not significant at a 95% confidence, therefore it, too, will not be significant at the same level of confidence.

The partial correlation coefficient table would suggest that there is no evidence for a relationship between free morphine at the post-mortem examination, and the two putative covariates, although the correlation matrix might suggest that there are. This is because the true nature of the relationships between the variables are masked by variables which are related to both covariates. When using correlation it is vital, if possible, to account for these 'hidden' relationships.

6.5 Partial correlation controlling for two or more covariates

Equation 14 is useful when the correlation between two covariates needs to be controlled for a third covariate, but what if there is more than one covariate which needs to be controlled for?

To calculate partial correlation coefficients controlling for more than a single variable it is necessary to perform some more advanced mathematical procedures. These can be undertaken using standard tools such as spreadsheets; further details on how to do this are given in Appendix G. The full correlation matrix is given below as Table 6.9, from which a partial correlation matrix has been calculated, given as Table 6.10. The significance of these partial correlations are listed in Table 6.11.

Table 6.9 Upper triangle of the correlation table for the variables featured in Table 6.5. The variables are morphine-3-glucuronide measured upon admission (M3G admission), morphine-3-glucuronide measured during post-mortem examination (M3G post-mortem), morphine-6-glucuronide measured upon admission (M6G admission), morphine-6-glucuronide measured during post-mortem examination (M6G post mortem), free morphine measured upon admission (FM admission) and free morphine measured during the post-mortem examination (FM post mortem). An approximate level of r for 95% significance is 0.44

Case	M3G admission	M3G post mortem	M6G admission	M6G post mortem	FM admission	FM post mortem
M3G admission	1.000	0.818	0.920	0.399	0.163	0.206
M3G post mortem	–	1.000	0.712	0.325	0.159	0.174
M6G admission	–	–	1.000	0.379	0.105	0.224
M6G post mortem	–	–	–	1.000	0.009	0.219
FM admission	–	–	–	–	1.000	0.538
FM post mortem	–	–	–	–	–	1.000

A level of correlation which could be considered significant for all values in Table 6.9 is approximately $r = 0.45$. This means that by using the correlations in a

Table 6.10 Upper triangle of the correlation table for the variables featured in Table 6.8. The variables definitions are the same as in Table 6.9

	M3G admission	M3G post mortem	M6G admission	M6G post mortem	FM admission	FM post mortem
M3G admission	−1.000	0.577	0.832	0.140	0.175	−0.124
M3G post mortem	−	−1.000	−0.178	0.002	0.012	0.015
M6G admission	−	−	−1.000	−0.013	−0.187	0.176
M6G post mortem	−	−	−	−1.000	−0.168	0.216
FM admission	−	−	−	−	−1.000	0.555
FM post mortem	−	−	−	−	−	−1.000

straightforward manner without controlling for inter-correlations in the data, there are four significant correlations. These are between morphine-3-glucuronide measured upon admission and morphine-3-glucuronide measured during post-mortem examination, and morphine-3-glucuronide measured upon admission morphine-6-glucuronide measured upon admission. There are also significant correlations between morphine-3-glucuronide measured during post-mortem examination and morphine-6-glucuronide measured upon admission, and free morphine measured upon admission and free morphine measured during the post-mortem examination.

If the correlations are controlled for the inter-correlations, then from Table 6.11 there are only three significant partial correlations. Those between morphine-3-glucuronide measured upon admission and morphine-3-glucuronide measured during post-mortem examination, morphine-3-glucuronide measured upon admission and morphine-6-glucuronide measured upon admission, and free morphine measured upon admission and free morphine measured during the post-mortem examination.

Table 6.11 Upper triangle of the significance table for the variables featured in Table 6.8. The variables definitions are the same as in Table 6.9.* indicates significance at a 95% confidence level

	M3G admission	M3G post mortem	M6G admission	M6G post mortem	FM admission	FM post mortem
M3G admission	−	*	*	−	−	−
M3G post mortem		−	−	−	−	−
M6G admission			−	−	−	−
M6G post mortem				−	−	−
FM admission					−	*
FM post mortem						−

The highly significant correlation between morphine-3-glucuronide measured during post-mortem examination and morphine-6-glucuronide measured upon admission is unexpected as it is difficult to conceive of how two different metabolites measured at two different times can be so highly related ($r = 0.712$). The same metabolite might be highly related when measured at different times because they are from a common precursor, or different metabolites at the same time, again because of the common precursor, but without postulating the effects of a common covariate a metabolite measured at one time should not be able to affect the concentration of a completely different metabolite measured at a different time.

If the effects of all the interrelations are accounted for by partial correlation then the partial correlation coefficient for the relationship becomes a non-significant $r = -0.178$.

We have just examined a small part of the data used by Gerostamoulos and Drummer (2000). The authors went on to examine the effect of location on the concentrations of metabolites. They sampled blood from subclavian and heart as well as the femoral location (given here in Tables 6.5 and Table 6.8) to look at the question of the redistribution of morphine and its metabolites about the human body in the post-mortem interval. They found no evidence of significant redistribution for any of the metabolites except for a minor, but non-significant, association with higher levels in the heart. They found little evidence for alteration with post-mortem interval.

Review questions

1. Estimate visually the nine linear correlation coefficients from the following graphs:

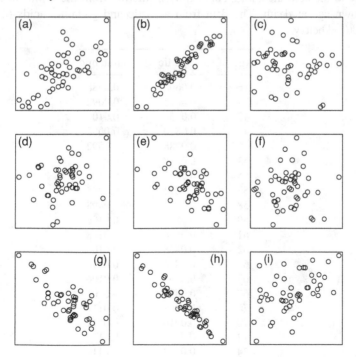

2. Levine *et al.* (2002) measured carboxyhaemoglobin saturation levels (COHb) in 42 cases where carboxyhaemoglobin had been a factor in the death of the individual through a variety of circumstances ranging from suicides to housefires. They measured

COHb in both heart and perpheral blood. The table below are these data from the first
10 cases from their Table 1.

Heart	Peripheral
11	14.0
12	4.2
14	12.0
16	16.0
18	20.0
18	33.0
20	19.0
23	24.0
24	38.0
26	29.0

One might expect to see a significant linear correlation between heart COHb and
perpheral COHb. Is this the case?

3. Ohtani *et al.* (2004) measured the D/L ratios for aspartic acid, glutamic acid and
alanine in the acid-insoluble, collagen-rich fraction from the femur in 21 cadavers
of known age at death. The data from aspartic and glutamic acids (Table 2) are
reproduced below.

Age	Aspartic	Glutamic
16	0.0608	0.0088
30	0.0674	0.0092
47	0.0758	0.0100
47	0.0820	0.0098
49	0.0788	0.0092
53	0.0848	0.0100
55	0.0832	0.0106
57	0.0824	0.0098
58	0.0828	0.0098
59	0.0832	0.0106
61	0.0826	0.0108
62	0.0838	0.0104
63	0.0874	0.0110
67	0.0864	0.0106
67	0.0870	0.0102
70	0.0860	0.0112
70	0.0910	0.0112
72	0.0912	0.0118
74	0.0932	0.0114
77	0.0916	0.0110
79	0.0956	0.0116

A plot of the D/L ratios of both amino acids suggests that both are highly related to age.

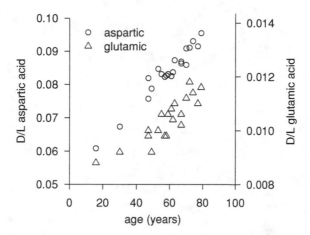

And indeed they are. The table below is the upper triangle of the correlation table for these three variables.[‡]

	Age	Aspartic	Glutamic
Age	1.00	0.97	0.88
Aspartic	–	1.00	0.86
Glutamic	–	–	1.00

In their paper Ohtani *et al.* (2004) conclude that the D/L ratio of aspartic acid is the best of the amino acid D/L ratios they examined. Given that D/L glutamic acid is also highly correlated with age is this correct?

[‡] Background theory suggests (Ohtani *et al.*, 2004) that a truly linear relationship is given by using $(1 + D/L)/(1 - D/L)$ with age. However, for this section of the curve there is an excellent approximation to a linear relationship. The difference between the correlation coefficients of age and D/L, and age and $(1 + D/L)/(1 - D/L)$ being found in the fourth or fifth decimal place.

7 Regression and calibration

In Chapter 5 we looked at measures of, and tests for, association between covariates where those covariates were nominal and/or ordinal. Chapter 6 dealt with the strength of relationship between covariates which are continuous, and the strength of relationship between covariates accounting for interdependence with other covariates. This Chapter will extend some of these ideas to the examination of the nature of the relationship between covariates which are continuous.

This is useful for a number of reasons, the primary one being that many variables are impossible to measure directly in a forensic context. Such variables may be age at death for human identification, post-mortem interval and time since discharge for a firearm. However, changes occur which are covariates of these immeasurables, things such as root dentine translucency (Solheim, 1989), the concentration of potassium ions in the vitreous humor (Munõz *et al.*, 2001), and as we have already seen, chemical residues in the barrels and chambers of firearms (Andrasko and Stähling, 1998). From measurements of these variables and knowledge of the exact nature of the relationship with the covariate which is not directly measurable, an estimate of the value of that covariate can be made. This process is called calibration; the establishment of the relationship from which a calibration can be taken is called modelling. We will concentrate on the simplest variety of mathematical modelling where the relationship between the two covariates is linear and monotonic.

7.1 Linear models

Munõz *et al.* (2001) published a table (Table 3) of values for post-mortem interval (PMI) and the concentration of vitreous potassium ions [K^+] for 164 cadavers from Spain. Table 7.1 is a sub-set of eight of these observations randomly selected from the original 164.

Table 7.1   Values for post-mortem interval (PMI) and
vitreous potassium ion concentration [K$^+$] for a sample
of eight cadavers from Munõz *et al.* (2001) reproduced
with permission

PMI	[K$^+$]
2.25	7.3
2.50	5.3
2.66	5.9
8.50	7.6
9.50	8.8
10.83	7.0
14.50	7.8
23.50	10.1

Figure 7.1 is a scatterplot of the data in Table 7.1.

From Figure 7.1 it is easy to imagine a single straight line going through the 'cloud' of xy points. This line would represent a linear model of PMI and [K$^+$]. Such a line is marked as the straight line on Figure 7.2.

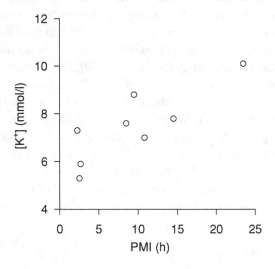

Figure 7.1   Scatterplot of post-mortem interval (PMI) and vitreous potassium concentration [K$^+$] for a sample of eight of the 164 cases examined by Munõz *et al.* (2001)

Any linear model which describes the relationship between two covariates may be described by two parameters, the values of which are termed coefficients. The first is the gradient or slope, the second is the intercept with the y axis. From Figure

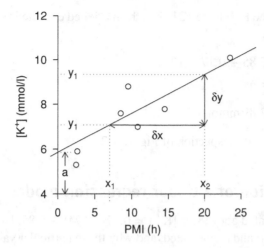

Figure 7.2 Linear model of PMI and [K$^+$]. Marked on this figure are the values x_1 and x_2, y_1 and y_2, and a, from which the parameters of the model can be calculated

7.2 the slope can be thought of as the change in y, or δy, divided by the change in x, or δx. It is very similar to the description of the gradient of a road as 1 in 20, or 1 in 5. For the slope of a road the 1 describes how far the road goes up vertically, the 20 or 5 being how long it takes in the horizontal direction to do this. When describing the gradient of a model we actually do the division to produce a single number, for the road example a gradient of 1 in 5 is $1/5 = 0.2$, or 20%, which is the more modern way of describing gradient on the roads of the United Kingdom. The gradient of a simple linear model is conventionally denoted b.

The same is true of the gradient of the model in Figure 7.2. A measure of the gradient is given by $\delta y / \delta x$. δy from the graph is $y_2 - y_1$. As $y_2 = 9.35$ and $y_1 = 7.07$, $\delta y = 2.28$. $x_2 = 20$, and $x_1 = 7$, so $\delta x = 13$. The gradient is $\delta y / \delta x = 2.28/13 = 0.17$.

An interpretation of this gradient of 0.17 is that for an increase of 1 h in PMI there is an increase of 0.17 mmol/l in vitreous [K$^+$]. This can be turned around to say that for every increase of 1 mmol/l in [K$^+$] there is an increase in $1/0.17 = 5.88$ h in PMI.

What of the coefficient a? a is marked on Figure 7.2, and is the intercept of the line with the y axis, as is the value of [K$^+$] when the PMI is zero. From Figure 7.2 this is 5.85.

A general form for a linear model is:

$$y = a + bx$$

where b is the gradient. In the specific case of PMI and [K$^+$]:

$$[K^+] = 0.17 \times PMI + 5.85 \tag{15}$$

Therefore, were the PMI to be 12 h then the modelled expected value of $[K^+]$ would be:

$$[K^+] = 5.85 + 0.17 \times 12$$

$$= 5.85 + 2.04$$

$$= 7.89 \, \text{mmol/l}$$

which is confirmed by inspection of Figure 7.2.

7.2 Calculation of a linear regression model

The model calculated above was $[K^+] = 0.17 \times \text{PMI} + 5.85$. How were these particular values for a and b calculated, and why those particular values? Why not any of the other line from the infinitude of possible lines which would be drawn through the data?

First we have to make an assumption that we need the 'best' line to describe the data. Then we need to define what a 'best' line might do. Usually in linear regression we calculate a 'best fit' model on the basis of minimizing the sum of squared errors in either the x or y direction. These errors are called residuals, and are the difference between the model and the true data.

Figure 7.3 is a detail of three of the points from Figure 7.2 showing these residuals. The objective of a *least squares regression* is to select the model which minimizes $\delta y_1^2 + \delta y_2^2 + \delta y_3^2 \ldots$.

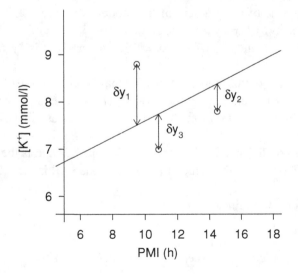

Figure 7.3 Detail of three points from Figure 7.2. Marked on the figure are the three residuals δx_1, δx_2 and δx_3

Without going into mathematical detail the estimate of the gradient b is:

$$b = \frac{S_{xy}}{S_{xx}} \tag{16}$$

where $S_{xx} = \sum(x_i - \bar{x})^2$ and $S_{xy} = \sum(x_i - \bar{x})(y_i - \bar{y})$. These two quantities should be quite familiar by now. The first (S_{xx}) is very similar to the variance of x, and is in fact equal to the numerator of the expression for variance from Equation 5 in Section 2.5. The second (S_{xy}) is the covariance between x and y seen in Section 6 being applied to the calculation of correlation coefficients.

We will omit further use of indices where the meaning is obvious, thus, x_i will be more simply written x, and y_i will be written y.

An estimate of the intercept a is given by:

$$a = \bar{y} - b\bar{x}.$$

Table 7.2 shows the calculations for these coefficients for the data in Table 7.1.

Table 7.2 Calculations for the regression y ([K$^+$]) fitted to x (PMI)

x	$x - \bar{x}$	$(x - \bar{x})^2$	y	$y - \bar{y}$	$(x - \bar{x})(y - \bar{y})$
9.50	0.22	0.05	8.8	1.33	0.29
14.50	5.22	27.25	7.8	0.32	1.70
10.83	1.55	2.40	7.0	−0.48	−0.74
2.25	−7.03	49.42	7.3	−0.18	1.23
2.66	−6.62	43.82	5.9	−1.58	10.43
8.50	−0.78	0.61	7.6	0.12	−0.10
23.5	14.22	202.21	10.1	2.62	37.33
2.50	−6.78	45.97	5.3	−2.18	14.75
$\bar{x} = 9.28$		$\sum 371.73$	$\bar{y} = 7.47$		$\sum 64.89$

From Table 7.2 $S_{xx} = \sum(x - \bar{x})^2 = 371.73$, and $S_{xy} = \sum(x - \bar{x})(y - \bar{y}) = 64.89$.

$$b = \frac{S_{xy}}{S_{xx}}$$

$$= \frac{64.89}{371.73}$$

$$= 0.1745$$

so the gradient b is 0.1745 for this linear fit. As $a = \bar{y} - b\bar{x}$, from Table 7.2, $\bar{x} = 9.28$ and $\bar{y} = 7.47$ and so $a = 7.47 - (0.1745 \times 9.28) = 5.85$.

7.3 Testing 'goodness of fit'

One of the first things we may wish to know about our model is whether it is a good fit to the data. Generally measures of this type are called 'goodness of fit' statistics.

Key to the calculation of the goodness of fit of any linear model is the notion of the sum of squared errors, and different sources of squared errors (Draper and Smith, 1981). Squared errors are the numerators used when calculating variance. Table 7.2 has two different sources of summed squared errors, that of x, $\sum(x - \bar{x})^2$ and of y, $\sum(y - \bar{y})^2$. There are other ways in which sums of squared errors can be envisaged, one of which is to imagine the summed differences between the points estimated from the regression, and the mean $\bar{y}$. This is known as the sum of squares due to regression. Another is the sum of squares between the true points of y and the estimates of those points. These two quantities when added together give the total sum of squared errors of y; so:

$$\sum(\hat{y} - \bar{y})^2 = \text{sum of squares due to the regression model}$$

$$\sum(y - \hat{y})^2 = \text{sum of squares about the regression model}$$

$$\sum(y - \bar{y})^2 = \text{total sum of squares}$$

where the estimate of y is denoted by the addition of an arrow over the letter, thus an estimate of y is written $\hat{y}$. Generally:

$$\sum(y - \bar{y})^2 = \sum(\hat{y} - \bar{y})^2 + \sum(y - \hat{y})^2$$

The proof of this is non-trivial and omitted. A suitable test statistic is:

$$F = \frac{\sum(\hat{y} - \bar{y})^2}{\frac{1}{df}\sum(y - \hat{y})^2} \tag{17}$$

where $df = n - 2$.

Because F is the ratio of the sum of squared residuals to the regression model to the sum of squared residuals about the regression model, i.e. the remainder of variability not accounted for by the model, then the larger the numerator relative to the denominator the more the model accounts for the relationship between the two covariates. Large values of F broadly mean that the model is more adequate than were small values to be obtained.

Taking values from Table 7.3, with $n = 8$, and $n - 2 = 6$, one obtains from Equation 17:

$$F = \frac{11.33}{\frac{1}{6} \times 4.92}$$

$$= 13.82$$

Table 7.3 Calculations for the 'goodness of fit' statistics the regression y ($[K^+]$) fitted to x (PMI)

x	y	$\hat{y}$	$y - \bar{y}$	$(y - \bar{y})^2$	$\hat{y} - \bar{y}$	$(\hat{y} - \bar{y})^2$	$y - \hat{y}$	$(y - \hat{y})^2$
9.50	8.8	7.51	1.33	1.76	0.04	0.00	1.29	1.66
14.50	7.8	8.39	0.32	0.11	0.91	0.83	−0.59	0.34
10.83	7.0	7.75	−0.48	0.23	0.27	0.07	−0.75	0.56
2.25	7.3	6.25	−0.18	0.03	−1.23	1.51	1.05	1.11
2.66	5.9	6.32	−1.58	2.48	−1.16	1.34	−0.42	0.18
8.50	7.6	7.34	0.12	0.02	−0.14	0.02	0.26	0.07
23.50	10.1	9.96	2.62	6.89	2.48	6.16	0.14	0.02
2.50	5.3	6.29	−2.18	4.73	−1.18	1.40	−0.99	0.98
$\bar{x} = 9.28$	$\bar{y} = 7.47$			$\sum 16.25$		$\sum 11.33$		$\sum 4.92$

This ratio is a value from another distribution, called the F-distribution. The F-distribution is a distribution associated with ratios of means. It has two parameters, the degrees of freedom for the numerator in the ratio and the degrees of freedom for the denominator in the ratio for the F in any simple linear regression the degrees of freedom for the numerator are 1, and the denominator $n - 2$, so a table is needed only for the second degrees of freedom at various standard levels of confidence. Such a table is given in Appendix F.

From Appendix F for 6 df at 5% significance the value of F is 5.99. The calculated value of F is 13.82 which is a more extreme difference than were the model not an adequate fit for these data, so we act as though the model is an adequate fit at the 5% level of significance. For 6 df the value of the F-distribution is at 13.75. The calculated value is only slightly greater than the tabulated value, so the model is just adequate at the 1% level of significance.

7.4 Testing coefficients *a* and *b*

The variance δ^2 for the model is estimated by the sum of squared deviations (s^2) divided by $n - 2$ degrees of freedom. This is best calculated as:

$$s^2 = \frac{S_{yy} - \dfrac{S_{xy}^2}{S_{xx}}}{n - 2}$$

The precision of a and b can be obtained by:

$$\text{ESE}(b) = \frac{s}{\sqrt{S_{xx}}}$$

$$\text{ESE}(a) = s\sqrt{\left(\frac{1}{n} + \frac{\bar{x}^2}{S_{xx}}\right)}$$

Taking values from from Table 7.2:

$$s^2 = \frac{16.25 - \frac{64.89^2}{371.72}}{8 - 2}$$

$$= \frac{16.25 - \frac{4210.71}{371.72}}{6}$$

$$= \frac{16.25 - 11.33}{6}$$

$$= 0.82,$$

$$s = 0.90.$$

The estimated standard error of b is:

$$\text{ESE}(b) = \frac{0.90}{\sqrt{371.73}}$$

$$= \frac{0.9}{19.28}$$

$$= 0.047$$

and for a

$$\text{ESE}(a) = 0.90\sqrt{\frac{1}{8} + \frac{9.28^2}{371.73}}$$

$$= 0.90\sqrt{\frac{1}{8} + \frac{86.12}{371.73}}$$

$$= 0.90\sqrt{0.36}$$

$$= 0.54.$$

A confidence interval for both a and b is calculated by using the appropriate value of the t-distribution with $n - 2$ degrees of freedom, so from Appendix D for a t-distribution with 6 df the 99% confidence level occurs at ± 3.707 standard errors. This means that a 99% confidence interval for $b = 0.1745 \pm 3.707 \times 0.047 = 0.1745 \pm 0.1742$, so the interval is 0.0002 to 0.3487. This interval is very close to zero at its lower limit which might provide evidence not to reject the hypothesis at 1% significance that the gradient of the model is zero, and that there is no systematic relationship between [K$^+$] and PMI. A similar confidence interval for a is $5.85 \pm 3.707 \times 0.54 = 5.85 \pm 2.0$ making the 99% confidence interval 3.85 to 7.85. This interval does not contain zero, so can be regarded as being evidence for the hypothesis that the intercept is non-zero.

7.5 Residuals

The main assumptions of simple linear regression are that the covariates are related in some meaningful way, and that they are linearly related. Both these requirements are tested to some degree by examination of a 'goodness of fit' statistic. However, there are other assumptions, such as the residuals must be normally distributed, implicit in the method. Violations of these assumptions can sometimes best be detected by what are known as residual plots. Residual plots are where the difference between values of y from the data, and the estimated values $\hat{y}$ are plotted against their respective x values.

A residual plot can show up a variety of violations of the assumptions of regression analysis. Figure 7.4 shows three possible problems which can be diagnosed from a residual plot. Figure 7.4(a) is a residual plot where all the assumptions of least squares regression modelling are met. There is no noticeable trend in the plot, and the spread of points in the y direction is uniform for all x. This is what we would expect to see if the assumptions of simple linear regression are met. Figure 7.4(b) is a residual plot where y is not linearly related to x. In this case $x \propto \log y$. There is a marked deviation curve, first down, then upwards, to these points through their x range. Other non-linear relationships will have different effects, but all will show some marked deviation from the ideal shown in Figure 7.4(a). Deviations from linearity between covariates will also be detectible in a scatterplot of the data. Figure 7.4(c) shows a residual plot from data in which the y values are autocorrelated. That is, the y value is dependent on covariate x, but is also dependent on other neighbouring y values. Here the residuals take the form of a sin function with respect to x, but other forms of autocorrelation will appear different. Depending on the nature of autocorrelation, various forms may appear exactly the same as the non-linearity seen in Figure 7.4(a), and can easily be confused with it. Ideally a test for autocorrelation would be used to differentiate between autocorrelated data, and non-linearly related covariates, but this is beyond the scope of this book. The final violation of assumption is where the distribution of the residual values varies with x and is termed heteroscedasticity. This is seen in Figure 7.4(d) where the residuals become larger as x increases producing a triangular pattern. This sort of pattern is often seen in data where one, or both, of the covariates have to take on positive values, because the data space is constrained in the region of low values.

Least squares regression analysis is robust to minor violations of the assumptions detailed in Figure 7.4, especially where a limited amount of heteroscedasticity is induced through a hard zero. Where the assumptions of regression are readily noticeable from a residual plot then there are methods available to correct for the problem. If the relationship between the covariates is non-linear then a non-linear regression may be used, or some simple transformation of the data made in a similar fashion to the way in which the log(time) was correlated with nitroglycerin to account for the

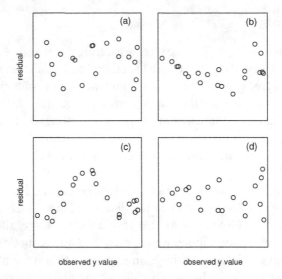

Figure 7.4 Illustrative residual plots showing violations of assumption. (a) is the residual plot from data which are linearly related, and represents a situation where all assumptions of linear regression are met. (b) is where the relationship between the two covariates is not linear. (c) is where the variable in the y direction is, where negative values are not possible, (d) is where the variance in y is not uniform throughout the range in x, or heteroscedastic

non-linearity in their relationship in Section 6.2. Usually non-linearity is explicable, and in many cases expected, from the background theory of the relationship between the covariates, and this will usually suggest some suitable model to use instead of a linear one. Autocorrelation is more difficult to account for and involves grouping of values and other advanced techniques. Fortunately it crops up less frequently as the autocorrelated variable has to be of a time series nature for the autocorrelation to have any meaning. Heteroscedasticity is seen more often, but unless one is trying to make estimates for values of the y variable it is often of little consequence. A standard set of methods for correcting highly heteroscedastic data are 'weighted' least squares regression methods, and are not covered any further here.

The residual plots from the regression of $[K^+]$ and PMI are in Figure 7.5. Figure 7.5(a) is the residual plot for the points for the sub-set of eight of the 164 points of Munõz *et al.* (2001). Here there is no evidence for anything other than a non-autocorrelated, heteroscedastic, linear relationship. However there are not many points on this plot, so it may not be too revealing about the extent and nature of any assumption violation for the relationship between $[K^+]$ and PMI. The residual plot for the full dataset is given in Figure 7.5(b), and, although there is the suggestion of some heteroscedasticity, the extent is not great. From Section 7.3 a linear model is an adequate fit, and this is confirmed by inspection of Figure 7.5(b), with no marked

an adequate fit, and this is confirmed by inspection of Figure 7.5(b), with no marked
or systematic deviation in the residuals. There is no evidence for autocorrelation in
either of the covariates.

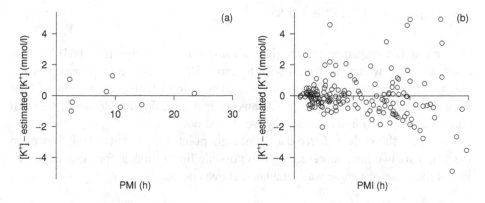

Figure 7.5   Residual plots for the regression of [K$^+$] and PMI. The values for the left hand graph
are for the reduced set from Table 7.3(a). The right graph (b) is a plot for all residuals from all
164 cases in Munõz *et al.* (2001), and include the eight data points from (a). The horizontal scale
is identical to (a) but the labels have been left out

The conclusion from the testing in Sections 7.3 and 7.4 is that there is a significant
linear relationship between [K$^+$] and PMI, with a non-zero gradient and non-zero
intercept with the y axis.

7.6 Calibration

We have now established that there is good evidence to suggest that there is a
linear relationship between [K$^+$] and PMI, and we know the parameters for this
relationship.

Why should this be of importance? Scientists are often in the position of not being
able to observe directly something which they may wish to know, however, they can
directly observe something related to the thing they wish to know, so, armed with
knowledge of the relationship between two covariates, an estimate can be made of
the desired value from direct observation of the covariate. This process is called
calibration.

In this instance it would be PMI which is not directly observable, however, a
measurement of [K$^+$] would be possible. From the regression model it should be
possible to make an estimate of PMI from the measurement of [K$^+$].

A linear calibration model

Fitting the values of $[K^+]$ to PMI using least squares regression gave us Equation 15, which is:

$$[K^+] = 0.17 \times PMI + 5.85$$

Notice this is an equation which gives a value for $[K^+]$ rather than PMI but it is a value of PMI which we would wish to know. Do we re-calculate the regression equation the other way around to produce an equation which gives a value of PMI for a direct observation of $[K^+]$? The answer is no, we do not. However, we shall continue to do so to find out just why we should not.

Figure 7.6 shows the reduced dataset of eight points for $[K^+]$ and PMI. Shown on the graph are two lines representing two possible linear models for these data. The line at the less steep angle was calculated above and is:

$$[K^+] = 0.17 \times PMI + 5.85 \tag{18}$$

From Figure 7.3 we can see that the fit is made by minimizing the residual error in the y direction, that is, by fitting $[K^+]$ to PMI. We can repeat this process, but

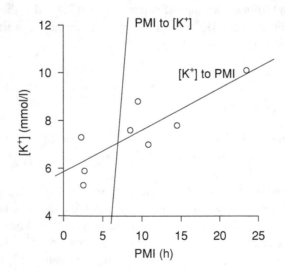

Figure 7.6 Detail of two possible regression models from Figure 7.3. The less steep of the two models is where the residuals are minimized in the y direction. This is where $[K^+]$ is fitted to PMI giving the model for the fit from Equation 18. The steeper of the two lines minimizes the residuals in the x direction, and is the regression of PMI fitted to $[K^+]$. The equation for this model is Equation 19

minimize the residuals in the x direction. From this we have the model

$$PMI = 4.00 \times [K^+] - 20.59 \qquad (19)$$

which is represented by the steeper of the two lines in Figure 7.3. Here we have fitted PMI to $[K^+]$.

If for the sub-set of eight points of these data we calculate estimates of PMI from the observation of $[K^+]$ using Equation 19, and then plot the difference between the true observation as y, and the estimate against the true observation on the x axis, we might expect to see a scatter of points varying randomly about zero with no particular trend observable. Unfortunately we do see a trend. Figure 7.7(a) is such a plot, the trend being clearer in Figure 7.7(b) which is the same plot for all 164 observations by Munõz et al. (2001).

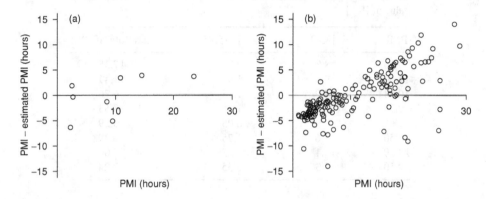

Figure 7.7 Residual plot of PMI minus estimates of PMI calculated from the regression model of PMI fitted to $[K^+]$ (Equation 19). (a) is for the subset of eight observations, a trend is noticeable, but more obvious in (b) which is the same plot for all 164 observations from the work of Munõz et al. (2001)

Here the trend gives systematically positive residuals for high values of PMI, and negative residuals for low values of PMI. This means that for high values of true PMI the true PMI minus the estimate of PMI is positive, suggesting that the estimate of PMI in this region is systematically lower than it should be. For low values of true PMI, PMI minus the estimate of PMI is negative, meaning that in this region of PMI the estimates tend to be systematically larger than the true values.

This is a bias in the estimates of PMI and is seen in estimates regardless of the nature of the observations where least squares regression modelling is used where the model is fitted the wrong way round. The magnitude of this bias is proportional to $1 - r^2$, where r is the correlation coefficient, and was noticed by Eisenhart (1939), the result being given in Draper and Smith (1988). A full explanation and proof is available in Aykroyd et al. (1997).

The question now has to be what can we do to avoid this bias? It turns out that we have already calculated a model which will avoid the bias, given in Equation 18. This has $[K^+]$ on the left-hand side, so needs rearranging to solve for PMI rather than $[K^+]$:

$$PMI = \frac{[K^+] - 5.85}{0.17} \qquad (20)$$

The calculation of estimates for PMI from $[K^+]$ is given in Table 7.4.

Table 7.4   Calculation of the estimates of PMI from Equation 20 for the sub-set of eight pairs of points from which the equation was calculated. The first column is PMI, the second column is $[K^+]$, the third column is calculated by taking the values in the second column and subtracting 5.85, and fourth column is calculated by taking the contents of the third and dividing by 0.17. This is the estimate of PMI from its corresponding value of $[K^+]$

PMI	$[K^+]$	$[K^+] - 5.85$	Estimate of PMI
9.50	8.8	2.95	17.35
14.50	7.8	1.95	11.47
10.83	7.0	1.15	6.76
2.25	7.3	1.45	8.53
2.66	5.9	0.05	0.29
8.50	7.6	1.75	10.29
23.50	10.1	4.25	25.00
2.50	5.3	−0.55	−3.24

The final estimate from Table 7.4 is −3.24 h. This is not in the range of possible values as PMI must be greater than zero. We shall leave this as it is for the moment, but if this value were to be reported it might be appropriate to changes the equation to zero.

The residuals for the estimates of PMI are plotted against PMI in Figure 7.8(a). There is less of a trend in this plot which is confirmed by examination of Figure 7.8(b) which features the same plot for all 164 pairs of points considered by Munõz *et al.* (2001).

The calibration model which fits $[K^+]$ to PMI adopted above was the model recommended by Munõz *et al.* (2001), and would avoid problems of bias, but what of other datasets, and what general principles can we deduce for instances where the covariates involved are not PMI and $[K^+]$?

In most instances where a linear calibration model is used the variable for which we wish to make estimates is an independent variable. An independent variable is one which is not dependent on its covariate. In the example above PMI is an independent variable.

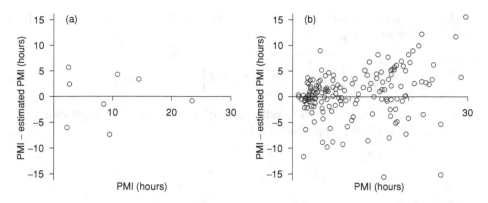

Figure 7.8 Residual plot of PMI minus estimates of PMI calculated from the regression model of [K$^+$] fitted to PMI (Equation 20). (a) is for the subset of eight observations, and (b) for all 164 observations from the work of Munõz *et al.* (2001). The residuals are, as might be expected, uniformly spread about the zero value with no noticeable bias as was seen in Figure 7.7(b)

The variable for which it is possible to make observations is often a dependent variable, that is, its value depends on the value of the independent variable. This is because of the notion of causation. PMI causes [K$^+$], but there is no way [K$^+$] can ever cause PMI. The same is true of many linearly related covariates. When using some chemical or physiological change to estimate age at death for a cadaver of unknown age, it is age which causes the chemical, or physiological change. The chemical or physiological change cannot in any sense cause a person's age when they happened to die. The same is true in the laboratory where in instrumental analysis one looks at the response of a measurement apparatus to a concentration. Here the concentration causes machine response, not the reverse. Essentially for all these simple situations where the variable for which we can make observations is dependent on the variable which we cannot directly measure, the dependent variable should be fitted to the independent variable, as we did above.

There are fewer instances where it is less obvious which way round to fit. For example, were skeletal measurements of the long bones being used to make estimates of stature for a cadaver of unknown stature, then which is the independent variable? Is it the long bone measurements, or stature? Stature is in a sense dependent on long bone measurements, so it might be more appropriate to fit stature to long bone length.

Calculation of a confidence interval for a point

The sorts of point estimates calculated above are only one element of an estimate of PMI from [K$^+$], some estimate of a confidence interval associated with any estimate of PMI would give an indication of the usefulness of the estimate itself.

An approximation for estimate of standard error for the point value of PMI is given (Miller and Miller, 1984):

$$S_{x0} = \frac{S_{y/x}}{b} \sqrt{\left\{ 1 + \frac{1}{n} + \frac{(y_0 - \bar{y})^2}{b^2 \sum (x - \bar{x})^2} \right\}} \tag{21}$$

where x is PMI, y is [K$^+$], and y_0 is the value of y for which a corresponding value of x is to be calculated. The value $S_{y/x}$ is:

$$S_{y/x} = \sqrt{\frac{\sum (y - \hat{y})^2}{n - 2}}$$

Equation 21 might look a little daunting, but in reality we have already calculated most of the quantities in it.

To calculate $S_{y/x}$ we need $\sum (y - \hat{y})^2$. The column sum from column 9 from Table 7.3 is $\sum (y - \hat{y})^2$ and is equal to 4.92. As the regression models we have calculated have been from a set of eight xy points then $n - 2 = 6$. So $S_{y/x} = \sqrt{0.82} = 0.91$.

Another quantity we need is $(x - \bar{x})^2$. The column sum for column 3 of Table 7.2 on is this quantity, and is equal to 371.73.

$b = 0.1745$ and from the fourth column of Table 7.2 $\bar{y} = 7.47$ and $n = 8$.

The first value of [K$^+$] from Table 7.4 is 8.8 mmol/l. Were this value to be observed then the corresponding calibrated value for PMI, from Equation 20, would be 17.35. The standard error associated with this point is:

$$S_{x0} = \frac{0.91}{0.1745} \sqrt{1 + \frac{1}{8} + \frac{(8.8 - 7.47)^2}{0.1745^2 \times 371.73}}$$

$$= 5.21 \sqrt{1 + \frac{1}{8} + \frac{1.33^2}{11.32}}$$

$$= 5.21 \sqrt{1 + \frac{1}{8} + 0.16}$$

$$= 5.21 \sqrt{1.285}$$

$$= 5.91$$

Table 7.5 is a table of this calculation for repeated all eight points.

To arrive at a suitable confidence interval the standard error of the estimate has to be multiplied by the appropriate value from the t-distribution for $n - 2$ degrees of freedom. That is:

$$x_0 = x_0 \pm t \times S_{x0}$$

From Appendix D at 95% confidence, and $n - 2 = 6$ df, the value of t is 2.447. The standard error for the first value in Table 7.5 is 5.91 and the point estimate for PMI is 17.35, so a 95% confidence interval is $17.35 \pm 5.91 \times 2.447 = 17.35 \pm 14.46$ or from 2.89 to 31.81 h. This means that for an observation of $[K^+]$ of 8.8 mmol/l there we have a 95% confidence interval of 2.89 to 31.81 h for the PMI.

Table 7.5 Calculation of standard errors for estimated PMI values

PMI	$[K^+]$	Estimate of PMI	SE of estimate
9.50	8.8	16.87	5.91
14.50	7.8	11.14	5.55
10.83	7.0	6.56	5.57
2.25	7.3	8.28	5.53
2.66	5.9	0.26	6.04
8.50	7.6	10.00	5.53
23.50	10.1	24.32	6.86
2.50	5.3	−3.18	6.48

The confidence interval cannot be interpreted as a probability distribution, that is, one should not say that there is a 95% probability that the PMI falls between 2.89 to 31.81 h, but it would be legitimate to say that there is a 95% confidence that the PMI lies between 2.89 to 31.81 h.

7.7 Points to remember

Regression and calibration are difficult subjects even for experienced statisticians. With the easy availability of statistical analysis software it is very tempting to use models which are inappropriate and overly complex. The solution is avoid using anything other than linear modelling unless background theory suggests a non-linear model is appropriate, or unless a linear model does not meet 'goodness of fit' criteria.

If the covariates really are related in some non-linear way usually some simple transformation, such as taking a log of one or both of the variables, will produce an adequate linear fit. Few sets of covariates will be related by some polynomial function, although most software packages will allow the user to fit high order polynomials.

If the data are multivariate, and a multivariate calibration is required, a multiple regression analysis from standard statistical software will not suffice. Multivariate calibration is a specific subject area within statistical science (Martens and Naes, 1989), and needs to be treated with care. A statistician will be required to guide the scientist through this sort of procedure.

From Figures 7.7(b) and 7.8(b) the way in which the model is fitted does require care and thought. Incorrect fitting, if used as a calibration model, can give very misleading estimated values. If in doubt plot the difference between estimates and true values against the true values for the training data, and see whether there is any trend in these. If there is any noticable trend then the assumptions, and fitting, of the model should be reconsidered.

This may be a little pedantic, but the values of [K$^+$] measured by Munõz *et al.* (2001) are in themselves estimates from a calibration experiment, and are subject to the same uncertainties in calibration as PMI. Munõz *et al.* (2001) used various instrumental methods to measure [K$^+$], and these tend to be highly accurate and precise. The error in measurement for [K$^+$] will be dwarfed by that of the variation between [K$^+$] and PMI, but for other analytical methods it may not be quite so clear and other calibration techniques would have to be adopted to account for instrumental error. In some circumstances it may be better to calibrate using the raw machine response to variation in the independent variable.

Finally, always plot covariates, residuals and residuals from calibration experiments. Good 'eyeball statistics' are more effective and give a better understanding of the relationships between variables than poorly understood and inappropriate tests.

Review questions

1. In their work on using vitreous humor as a suitable site from which to test for benzodiazepines during post-mortem drug analysis Scott and Oliver (2001) measured temazepam, diazepam and desmethyldiazepam in the blood, and vitreous humor of 17 cadavers. For diazepam they give the following table reproduced with permission:

Vitreous humor (mg/l)	Blood (mg/l)
0.18	Nd
1.98	0.63
0.44	0.39
1.01	0.74
0.47	0.47
0.15	0.15
0.29	Nd
0.55	Nd
Nd	0.62
0.45	0.07
0.03	0.01
0.27	0.10
Nd	Nd
0.08	0.10
1.51	1.25
Nd	Nd
2.62	2.48

where Nd means not detected.

Scott and Oliver (2001) say that 'The transport of drugs across the blood vitreous humor barrier is limited by the lipid solubility of . . .'.

Scott and Oliver (2001) used linear regression modelling on these data, and made the claim that gradient of the regression is different from 1 suggesting that the concentration of diazepam in blood is higher than in vitreous humor.

(a) Is this claim true?
(b) Is the concentration of diazepam seen in vitreous humor a good indicator of blood diazepam concentration?

2. A recent immigrant to Germany shot and killed three women in a Berlin fitness centre. He claimed he should not get a life sentence in prison because he was under 22 years of age at the time of the murders. His passport suggested that he was over 22 at that time, however he claimed he had lied to German immigration officials upon entry to Germany. In an attempt to resolve the issue over the offender's age various biometric measures of age were made, which included the removal of a tooth. The tooth was extracted some 9 months after the offence took place.

Gillard et al. (1990) used measurements of the %D-aspartic acid from tooth dentinal collagen from first premolars as a measure of adult human age at death. Here is a sub-set of the data given by Gillard et al. (1990) and is reproduced with permission.

age (years)	% D-aspartic acid
9	1.13
10	1.10
11	1.11
12	1.10
13	1.24
14	1.31
33	2.25
39	2.54
52	2.93
65	3.40
69	4.55

If the tooth from the offender were a first premolar, and the %D-aspartic acid from the tooth found to be 2.01, and were the Gillard et al. (1990) dataset used as a calibration set for age, would the investigators stand any chance of telling whether the offender was under 22 at the time of the murders?

The following summary statistics are available:

$\bar{x}$	29.73
$\bar{y}$	2.06
$\sum(x - \bar{x})(y - \bar{y})$	268.03
$\sum(x - \bar{x})^2$	5390.15
$\sum(\hat{y} - \bar{x})^2$	13.28
$\sum(y - \hat{x})^2$	0.54

8

Evidence evaluation

The preceding chapters have been concerned with standard statistical methods of data analysis. Over the century or so since the methods of probability were applied to enumerated data, many different types of test and methods of analysis have been devised and used in all fields of scientific knowledge where precise measurement is a feature. Many of these tests and statistical techniques are applicable, and widely available to laboratory based science, however, there is a body of statistical science which is unique to the forensic sciences. The remainder of this book is devoted to an exploration of the aims, theoretical bases for, and practical methods of application for a set of statistical thinking called evidence evaluation.

One of the most pressing questions for anyone called upon to examine forensic evidence is *what do these data mean?* That is, what are these data suggesting in relation to a set of propositions which may be put forward by a court? This is a question that statisticians have been working on with some success since the late 1970s, for which there is a substantial body of theoretical and practical knowledge.

This chapter will attempt to place the fundamental concepts of modern statistically based evidence evaluation into an everyday context without a mathematical derivation. More mathematical parts will be reserved for later chapters.

8.1 Verbal statements of evidential value

It is common to evaluate forensic evidence simply by reporting the features of a case, and whether, in the experience of the forensic scientist, the evidence would have occurred as a result of an offence committed on the part of the suspect. Epistemologically forensic science is at its most certain when it can exclude suspects. For instance, a non-matching DNA profile in a rape case will effectively remove with great certainty an individual from suspicion. Unfortunately exclusions, although vital, rarely come to court, as courts seldom try those who are known to be innocent.

Introduction to Statistics for Forensic Scientists   David Lucy
© 2005 John Wiley & Sons, Ltd.

It is unfortunate that forensic science is least certain when in some senses it needs to be most certain.

A phrase such as 'consistent with' is often used to denote some unquantified positive evidential value. However it is a very weak statement of evidential value. In science 'is consistent with' means that the evidence has failed to refute some proposition. For scientists a tested, but unrefuted hypothesis, is one which can be considered provisionally true (Popper, 1962). Unfortunately, amongst lay persons, 'is consistent with' can be taken as offering some higher level of support for the proposition (Robertson and Vignaux, 1995) than the phrase demands at some logical level. Another phrase which has been used is 'does not exclude', which is not a statement of unquantified positive support at all, but simply a statement of lack of negative support. Sometimes, due to the ambiguous and unquantifiable nature of some evidence types, all that can be said is that the evidence has failed to exclude some proposition, however, any statement to this effect is logically very weak in support of the converse proposition. Most forensic scientists will try to provide some idea of the extent to which they think the evidence provides positive support for some proposition, even if it is just in terms of a subjective probability, based on experience, of seeing the observations which form the source of the evidence.

It is the whole area of positive support for propositions with which statistical evaluation of evidence is concerned.

8.2 Evidence types

Were a suspect to possess a particular observable characteristic, let us for convenience say a brown woollen pullover, and it is known that the individual who committed some specific offence possesses the same observable characteristic, then that characteristic would form in some sense a piece of evidence which supports a link between the suspect and the offender.

Some classes of characteristic can fail to undermine positive evidence linking a suspect to a criminal offence. For instance, were it known that the offender had a pair of black leather gloves in addition to the brown pullover, and the suspect did not have a pair of black leather gloves, but had a brown pullover, then the absence of leather gloves would not detract from the evidential value of the brown pullover.

Other classes of observable characteristics can eliminate people. For instance, were it known the offender had a tattoo on his/her left hand, and the suspect did not have such a tattoo, then the evidence of a tattoo would effectively exclude the suspect from further consideration.

The evidence types listed above are classifiable into two categories, that where the evidence is an integral part of the offender, and suspect, and that where it is not. Failure of a suspect's DNA profile to match that of an offender excludes that suspect from further consideration as the offender in the same way that the absence of a tattoo would exclude a suspect.[†] However, the absence of a brown pullover would not safely exclude a suspect in the same way as would a non-matching DNA profile.

For evidence types which are an intrinsic property of the offender and suspect, such as a tattoo or DNA, does possession of the characteristic mean that the suspect is the offender? Not necessarily. In the case of it being known that an offender possesses a tattoo on the left hand, the suspect who has a similar feature might be only one of many individuals with a tattoo on the left hand.

DNA evidence, although very compelling, is the same in that a suspect matching the profile of an offender may be one of a set, albeit a very small set, of individuals who share that profile.

DNA profiles and tattoos can exclude suspects from consideration on the basis of negative observations, portable evidence types such as brown pullovers and gloves cannot. But what if suspect and offender share characteristics? To what extent should one believe in the guilt or innocence of a suspect on the basis they share some indistinguishable item of clothing, or have some indistinguishable immutable characteristic in common.

8.3 The value of evidence

Let us imagine that a criminal offence has been committed, and that an eyewitness says the offender had a tattoo on his/her left hand. Forensic scientists say that the offender wore a brown pullover based upon the analysis of fibres found at the crimescene. From a population of possible suspects numbering 100 000 it is known that 100 people have a tattoo on their left hand, and that 10 000 people possess brown pullovers. A suspect has been detained on grounds unrelated to the evidence who fits the description of possessing a brown pullover, and a tattoo on the left hand.

From these numbers it is a matter of intuition that the observation of a tattoo on the left hand is more compelling as evidence for the guilt of the suspect than the fact that the suspect possesses a brown pullover. The question is by how much does the tattoo support the proportion that the suspect is offender, and why?

An answer to this might be to examine the probability of guilt given the observation that the suspect possesses a tattoo on the left hand, and a brown pullover respectively. In the first case there are 100 people in the population who have tattoos on their left hands and the offender is one of these people, so with no other information there is a probability of 1/100 that the suspect is the offender. Likewise for the brown pullover, there are 10 000 people with brown pullovers in the population, the offender is one of these 10 000, therefore with no other information there is a probability of 1/10 000 that the suspect is the offender.

There are some problems with the answers given above. Is the 1/100 figure high or low? If one were expecting to win at some game where the probability of success

---

[†] Modern surgical techniques will remove a tattoo without scarring, but these are costly and take a long time.

is 1/100 one would not be too disappointed at failure. Putting it into the context of betting, the evidence of a tattoo on the left hand is not very persuasive. The brown pullover is of even less evidential worth when examined like this.

Another problem with the approach above is sensitivity to the size of the total population. If the population were 1 000 000, and the proportion of people with similar tattoos remains unchanged relative to the potential suspect population size, there would be 1000 people with a tattoo on their left hand. The offender must be one of these, therefore with no other knowledge there is a probability of 1/1000 of the suspect being the offender.

However, it is counter-intuitive that the persuasive value of a piece of evidence is any less just because it comes from a larger population of potential suspects. If that were true it would mean that no matter how rare a piece of evidence is amongst the population of potential suspects, simply increasing the size of the population would reduce the value of that piece of evidence. For instance a piece of evidence, possibly some genetic marker, which may occur with the *same frequency* in the populations of the People's Republic of China and the United Kingdom, would, in the United Kingdom have a probative value of 21 times that of the same evidence in the People's Republic of China, as the population of the People's Republic of China is 1265 million, and the population of the United Kingdom is only 60 million. This obviously cannot be true.

A further problem is that in these calculations we are assessing the probability of the suspect being the offender, effectively the probability of guilt given the evidence. This is not the same as making some comment on the strength of the evidence; it is making a statement about the propositions of guilt or innocence. Ideally there should be some measure of evidential strength which tells us about the strength of the evidence in support of a proposition of guilt or innocence, without it actually telling us how likely or unlikely the proposition of guilt or innocence itself is. That is, ideally there should be a way of *distilling* the effect of the evidence which would be related to the persuasive power of the evidence in relation to the legal questions, and independent of other philosophical and epistemological concerns.

One way of doing this is to think about the probability of guilt before we are introduced to the evidence, and compare this with the probability of guilt after we know what the evidence is. In this way we might be able to isolate the effect of the evidence in the light of the propositions of guilt or innocence.

Were a population to have 100 000 members, then were we to assume that each person in it were equally likely to be guilty of the offence as each other person, then before any evidence is known the probability of each person being the offender would be 1/100 000. As calculated above, if there are 100 people with tattoos on their left hands, and the offender must be one of these, then the probability of a suspect selected at random from the population matching the known offender characteristic is 1/100. Therefore the evidence has taken us from thinking that there is a 1/100 000 probability to a 1/100 probability, that is, a 1000-fold increase in the probability of the suspect's guilt.

This increase of 1000 fold can be seen as the effect that the evidence has on our calculated probability of the suspect being the offender. We started with an opinion that the offender could be any of 100 000 individuals, and it has been narrowed down to any of 100 individuals by use of this evidence. This increase in belief makes the evidence quite valuable.

The same reasoning can be applied to the evidence of the brown pullover. Initially if it is assumed each individual in the population is equally likely to be the offender there is a 1/100 000 probability that the suspect is guilty. After the brown pullover has been observed as a characteristic of the suspect, and the offender must be one of these 10 000 individuals, there is a 1/10 000 probability the suspect is the offender. This gives a 10-fold increase in the probability of the suspect's guilt, and again this could be interpreted as the effect the evidence is having on our degree of belief.

What if the starting population was of 1 000 000 potential suspects? Were the proportion of individuals with tattoos on the left hand the same as in the case where there were only 10 000 in the population, then there would be 1000 individuals with tattoos on the left hand. Before the evidence of the tattoo on the left hand is brought into play we suspect each member of the population equally, giving a 1/1 000 000 probability that the individual who is under suspicion is the offender. After the tattoo has been observed then the probability that the suspect is the offender has risen to 1/1000, which is a 1000-fold increase, the same as where we had the same proportion of tattooed individuals, but a smaller population of potential suspects.

Here we have an approach which measures just the effect of evidence and is solely affected by the numbers of individuals who share the characteristic under consideration in the population. The measure of evidential weight here is invariant to the absolute size of the population from which the suspect and offender may be drawn.

Unfortunately it is difficult to justify using this approach as it stands because we have to make an explicit assumption in the first instance that each individual in the population is equally likely to be the offender, something which simply is not true. We then have to make the explicit assumption when the evidence has been observed that each individual from the population sharing the characteristic which forms the evidence is equally likely to be the offender. Again this is unwarrantable, and despite this approach being invariant to the size of population one still needs to know the size of the population.

Is there some measure, analogous to the analysis above, which measures the value of the evidence by some increase in support for a proposition, but avoids the problems of population specification?

We may not be sure of the absolute population size of potential suspects, and may be unwilling to make assumptions about suspecting each member of the population equally, but we may be reasonably certain of the frequency of occurrence of the characteristic which forms the evidence. One way in which this may be considered is to interpret this frequency in terms of the question of the guilt, or innocence of the suspect.

So what is this frequency? In the original population we had 100 000 people, 100 of whom had tattoos on their left hands. Only one of the 100 000 was the offender, and the tattoo helped to narrow that down to one of 100 with tattoos on the left hand. The frequency of 100 in 100 000, or 0.001, refers to just the frequency of finding a tattoo on the left hand. However, 99 999 of the 100 000 population are innocent, as are 99 of those with tattoos on their left hands. Of non-offenders the frequency of finding a tattoo on the left hand is 99 in 99 999 = 0.00099 ≈ 0.001. The probability of finding an individual in the population with a tattoo on their left hand is 0.001, and we can also say that the the probability of observing a tattoo on the left hand *given* that the person is innocent of the offence is 0.00099 ≈ 0.001.

This is not the figure of 1000 which so easily described the effect of the evidence as an increase in probability of having selected the offender. So how do we get back to an intuitive figure which measures the persuasive power of the evidence alone?

We have calculated the probability of seeing the evidence, in this case a tattoo on the left hand, were the suspect not the offender; this is 0.00099 ≈ 0.001. What is the probability of seeing that same evidence if the suspect is the offender? We know that the offender possessed a tattoo on their left hand, as does the suspect, so if the offender is the suspect, then the probability of that evidence is 1, or inevitable. This is because the suspect has only one left hand, the suspect's left hand has a tattoo, therefore, were the suspect the offender, the offender would also have a tattoo on their left hand.

How does this help us? We have calculated the probability of seeing the evidence were the suspect the offender, which is 1, and we have calculated the probability of the evidence were the suspect not the offender, which is ≈0.001. The value of 1 is 1000 times greater than 0.001, so the probability of the evidence is ≈1000 times greater were the suspect the offender, than were the suspect not the offender. Therefore, with the evidence, one could say there is a 1000-fold increase in support of the proposition that the suspect is the offender over the proposition that the suspect is not the offender. This increase in support being due to the introduction of the evidence.

The figure of a 1000-fold increase is the same as when we calculated the effect of the evidence by considering the probabilities of the suspect's guilt before and after the evidence came into play. We have simply calculated the effect that the evidence is having upon our belief in a similar way, but using different data.

From the examples given above it might be thought that the evaluation of the effect of a particular piece of evidence is simply a matter of finding the frequency of the observable in the population of interest. If this were true then it might be thought unnecessary to evaluate the probability of observing the evidence were the suspect the offender. This would only be true if it were inevitable that the evidence from the suspect would match that from the offender were the suspect truly the offender. In many cases this is true, but not always, so we do need some system for evidence evaluation which is flexible enough to take this into account.

Take, for instance, the example above of the brown pullover. We have seen how to evaluate the observation of such an item, and how it is of less evidential value than the observation of a tattoo on the left hand because it occurs with a greater frequency in the population as a whole. However, what if brown pullovers and tattoos on the left hand were to occur with an equal frequency in the population? Our formulation above would suggest they would be of equal evidential value. But would this be right? Were these pieces of evidence presented in a court during criminal proceedings it might be that the observation of a tattoo would carry a greater weight than the observation of a brown pullover. This is because, as discussed earlier in this chapter, the brown pullover is an easily portable piece of evidence. Unlike a tattoo which cannot be removed at short notice, it is not inevitable that an offender will wear a brown pullover, or indeed any pullover if they possess one, whilst committing an offence.

So how does one evaluate this type of portable evidence? One needs an evaluation of the probability of the evidence were the suspect the offender. The evidence is the observation of a brown pullover associated with the offender, and associated with the suspect, which could be taken to be the frequency of brown pullovers in the suspect's wardrobe. That is, were the suspect to possess five pullovers, two of which were brown, then the probability of observing a brown pullover if the suspect were the offender would be 2/5.

Putting these components together we have the probability of seeing the evidence were the suspect the offender, which is 2/5, divided by the probability of observing a brown pullover given the suspect is not the offender, which, as calculated earlier, is 9999/99,999. This evaluates to ≈ 4, which is less than the ≈ 10 were some evidence with the same frequency as the brown pullover in the population an immutable part of the suspect, the reduction being due to the property of portability of an article of clothing.

The 9999/99,999 probability of observing a brown pullover given that the suspect is not the offender is fairly clear cut, and based upon the frequency of brown pullovers in the general population. However, the 2/5 probability of the suspect choosing a brown pullover is something of a subjective choice. It could be that one of the other pullovers belonging to the suspect is bright pink in colour, and simply would not be suitable as apparel for this particular offence, in which case the selection of a brown pullover would be a 2/4 event, as there are only four suitable pullovers from which to choose. On the other hand it might be considered that all suitable clothing for the torso should be amongst the set from which the pullover might be selected, in which case were the suspect's wardrobe to contain five suitable jackets as well as the four pullovers then the probability would be 2/9.

This element of uncertainty and indecision is a constant feature of the evaluation of evidence and is easier to resolve in some cases than in others. For instance, in the example of both the offender and suspect having a tattoo on the left hand then there is very little problem as the probability of the suspect having a tattoo were the suspect the offender would be one as the tattoo is to all practical purposes an immutable characteristic of both offender and suspect.

Modern notions of the statistical evaluation of evidence revolve around the idea that the value of evidence is linked to the magnitude of the change in knowledge that the evidence brings by being considered. It is not an evaluation of the probability of a proposition such as 'the suspect is guilty', or the 'suspect is innocent'. Instead evidence evaluation is about the 'probability of evidence' in the light of competing hypotheses. This allows the scientist to confine their statements and analysis to their field of expertise, namely the evidence, and not to comment on the ultimate issue of whether a suspect committed a particular crime or not.

It also allows the investigator to analyse rationally their beliefs as to the relative strengths and weakness of specific evidence types. For instance, most people would agree that the observation of a tattoo on the left hand is of a greater probative value than the observation of a brown woollen pullover, but might not necessarily be able to frame this intuition in terms of the relative frequencies of the observations, and the number of similar items which are 'fit for purpose' in the suspect's possession. The approach outlined above will be put onto a more sound mathematical basis in Section 9.2.

8.4 Significance testing and evidence evaluation

From Section 4.5 it might be thought that the problem of establishing a probability for one object coming from another object based upon a series of measurements had been solved. For instance, were a crime committed and some glass broken, then a suspect might be found with glass fragments on their clothing. It might be thought that examination of the glass fragments from the scene (*control*), and those from the suspect (*recovered*) if measured in a suitable way and the means of those measurements t-tested, might lead to a confidence being attached to them being from the same source. Unfortunately this would be entirely misleading.

To illustrate why, imagine two crimes, and two sets of glass. One of the buildings is on a medium density housing estate with a well-known brand of double glazing units. The other is Durham Cathedral[‡], with 14th century stained glass being the broken pane. Were this the case, and the suspect in each case found to have glass fragments from these types of windows on their clothing, then no matter how close a match it follows intuition that the glass from the housing estate will be of a lesser probative value than that from the Cathedral.

The reason is that glass from similar units in the housing estate can be found in hundreds of thousands of windows throughout Britain, whereas 14th century stained glass can only be found in a few dozens of windows. Put another way, the Cathedral glass is much rarer than the sealed unit double glazing glass, consequently the chances of finding it in innocent contact with a suspect are far lower than that for the double glazing glass.

In other words the t-testing seen in Section 4.5 will only compare means of samples to see if they could have come from a population with the same mean, not

---

[‡] Durham is a small city in the north of England with a particularly fine Gothic cathedral.

whether the control and recovered fragments are from the same pane. To use a test, such as the *t*-test, in this way would be to commit an error in interpretation called the *different levels* error (Section 13.2.1). That is where inferences are made about the origin of any object based solely on similarities from the compositional level in a hierarchy of possible similarities. To make legitimate probabilistic inferences about the connection between any two objects requires not only some measure of similarity in characteristics, but also how many other objects from a wider population of objects share those characteristics. Put simply *proximity of observation does not by necessity equal identity between objects.*

This is one of the reasons why we cannot use standard statistical tests to deduce the probability, or some significance, or confidence level, for the 'match' between two objects. A statement of reporting a 'match' is more or less meaningless unless it is accompanied by some statement of how often a similar 'match' could be seen.

Does this mean that procedures such as *t*-testing are useless for forensic scientists? It does not; it all depends on what one is expecting them to do. If in the laboratory you are interested in the differences between sets of measurements from similar things, and whether you can distinguish between them on the basis of these measurements, then significance testing is entirely appropriate. You could even use something such as a *t*-test as a basis to exclude one set of measurements from a recovered object as having been derived from a control object due to the dissimilarity in measurement, and this would be quite a powerful statement, although other more suitable methods exist. What you cannot do with some standard significance test is interpret what any measured similarity means. Standard statistical tests just do not do that.

Review Questions

1. A road traffic accident has occurred in which a person was injured. The driver of one of the vehicles left the scene before the arrival of the police and left no details at the accident scene. The only reliable eye-witness says that the car of the missing driver was silver in colour. Silver paint has been found at the scene and a number of properties measured, and a suspect has been identified who has a silver Ford Focus. The paint examiner says that they cannot exclude the suspect's Ford Focus from being the vehicle which left the paint trace at the accident scene. How persuasive is this evidence that the suspect's car is that involved in the accident? (Non-numeric answer required).

2. A similar same situation as to that found in the question above, except this time the colour of the paint found at the scene is vivid lime green. The suspect has a vivid lime green Ford Focus, and the paint examiner again cannot exclude the suspect's car from being that which left the paint at the accident scene. How persuasive is the paint evidence that the suspect's car was involved in the accident? (Non-numeric answer required).

9 Conditional probability and Bayes' theorem

In Section 3.1 we examined probabilities for events which were independent. Independence implied that to calculate the probabilities for joint events (the coincidence of two or more events) the probabilities for the single events could be multiplied. In this chapter, the more common case, events are not thought to be independent, will be examined. This will eventually lead to the same idea for evidence evaluation as that seen in Section 8.3, although a more mathematical approach will be taken.

9.1 Conditional probability

According to Lee (2004, p. 5) all probabilities are conditional probabilities, that is, the probability of a coin landing with the heads face uppermost being 0.5 is conditional on it being a fair coin. As we saw in Section 3.1.4, even simple die throwing systems can force us to think explicitly in terms of conditional probabilities, so it might be expected that consideration of empirical data would entail the further exploration of conditional probability.

Rogers *et al.* (2000) give an analysis which uses the *rhomboid fossa* as an indicator of the sex of unknown skeletalized human remains. The rhomboid fossa is a groove which sometimes occurs on one end of the clavicle as a result of the attachment of the rhomboid ligament, and on skeletalized remains is more frequent in males than females.

The contingency table[†] shown in Table 9.1 has been reconstructed from Rogers *et al.* (2000, Table 2[‡]), and is simply a count of how many individuals fall in each

---

[†] Sometimes called a cross table.
[‡] Rogers *et al.* (2000) give counts for left and right clavicle separately; they give no indication about those possessing left and right rhomboid fossas. During the adaptation of their data for this illustration it has been assumed that there were no skeletons with both left and right clavicles affected. This assumption is probably untrue, but does not affect the data for the purposes of illustration.

Introduction to Statistics for Forensic Scientists   David Lucy
© 2005 John Wiley & Sons, Ltd.

Table 9.1 Cross-tabulation of sex and presence and absence of a rhomboid fossa. Reproduced with permission

	present	absent	row sum
male	155	76	231
female	12	101	113
column sum	167	177	344

category, for example, the authors counted 155 male skeletons with a rhomboid fossa, and 101 female skeletons without one. The bottom row and right-hand column are simply sums of the corresponding row and column, and correspond to total numbers of objects; for instance, reading the first entry in the right-hand column there were 231 male skeletons observed, and the second entry in the bottom row there were 177 skeletons without a rhomboid fossa observed.

The grand total in the bottom right-hand corner is the total number of skeletons observed, and equals 344. This is used to calculate some of the probabilities. Table 9.2 is a table of the probabilities for the joint event $Pr(S_j$ and $R_i)$ where S_j is the event of being S_m (male) or S_f, (female), and R_i is the event of having (R_p) a rhomboid fossa, or not having (R_a), a rhomboid fossa.

Table 9.2 Joint probabilities for sex and the presence and absence of a rhomboid fossa

$Pr(S_j$ and $R_i)$	present	absent	$Pr(S_j)$
male	0.45	0.22	0.67
female	0.03	0.30	0.33
$Pr(R_i)$	0.48	0.52	1.00

These probabilities are calculated by simply dividing every value in Table 9.1 by the grand total of 344, that is 155 males with a rhomboid fossa divided by 344 individuals inspected give 0.45 or 45% of 344 individuals inspected were male *and* had a rhomboid fossa. The same can be said of the 101 female skeletons examined, that is, $101/344 = 0.30 = 30\%$ of 344 skeletons were female *and did not* have a rhomboid fossa.

These are interpretable as probabilities in the same way as were the Δ^9-THC concentrations in marijuana seizures in Talk 3. One could make a proposition that a randomly selected individual skeleton from the 344 would have a 45% probability of being male and having a rhomboid fossa, and a 29% probability of being female and not having a rhomboid fossa.

The right-hand column of Table 9.2 tells us the probability of any one of the 344 skeletons examined being from a man or woman, that is $Pr(S_m) = 0.67 = 67\%$ male and $Pr(S_f) = 0.33 = 33\%$.

The bottom row tells us the probability of any randomly selected individual from the 344 having a rhomboid fossa or not, that is $\Pr(R_p) = 0.48 = 48\%$ and $\Pr(R_a) = 0.52 = 52\%$.

These last two sets of probabilities can be called unconditional probabilities[§], that is, in the sample the probability of selecting at random an individual without a rhomboid fossa is 0.52, or the probability of selecting a female is 0.33 without any other conditions. They are not unconditional in any absolute sense, but are not explicitly conditioned on any other factors in the dataset.

However, there is another sort of probability which can be calculated other than the joint probabilities and the unconditional probabilities: these are the conditional probabilities.

With a conditional probability we are asking the question: if we know an individual is a male, what is the probability they have a rhomboid fossa? Or conversely, if the skeleton does not have a rhomboid fossa, what is the probability that the skeleton came from a female? This question is the same sort of question we came across in Section 3.1.4 with dice where the event of throwing an odd number which was greater than three, but framed in a different way.

From Table 9.1 there are 231 males, of whom 155 have a rhomboid fossa, 76 do not, so the probability of having a rhomboid fossa given that the skeleton is male is $155/231 = 0.67 = 67\%$, or in notation $\Pr(R_p|S_m) = 0.67$, where the vertical line means *conditioned on*, or *given*. The terms given and conditioned on can be considered synonymous in probability theory.

Similarly the probability of observing the absence of a rhomboid fossa given the skeleton comes from a male is $76/231 = 0.33 = 33\%$.

For females $\Pr(R_p|S_f) = 0.11$ and $\Pr(R_a|S_f) = 0.89$. This is summarized in Table 9.3.

Table 9.3 Probability the presence or absence of a rhomboid fossa given the sex of the individual

$\Pr(R_i \mid S_j)$	present (R_p)	absent (R_a)
male (S_m)	0.67	0.33
female (S_f)	0.11	0.89

From Table 9.1 it is also possible to consider the values appearing in the columns. From this we have the converse conditional probability from those in Table 9.3. The question is now: what is the probability of observing a skeleton with a rhomboid fossa and finding that they are female, or what is the probability of a female skeleton possession a rhomboid fossa? We know there are 167 skeletons with rhomboid fossae, 12 of which are female, and 155 being male, so the probability is $12/167 =$

[§] They are also sometimes called marginal probabilities, or marginals.

$0.07 = 7\%$. The probability of a skleleton with a rhomboid fossa being male is $155/167 = 0.93 = 93\%$.

Likewise $\Pr(S_f \mid R_a) = 101/177 = 0.57 = 57\%$ and is the probability of a skeleton being female *given* lack of a rhomboid fossa, and $\Pr(S_m \mid R_a) = 76/177 = 0.43 = 43\%$ is the probability of the skeleton being male given they have no rhomboid fossa. The conditional probability $\Pr(S_j \mid R_i)$ is summarized in Table 9.4.

Table 9.4   Probability of the sex of an individual given the presence or absence of a rhomboid fossa

$\Pr(S_j \mid R_i)$	present (R_p)	absent (R_a)
male (S_m)	0.93	0.43
female (S_f)	0.07	0.57

If a skeleton from the sample is observed to possess a rhomboid fossa then it is perfectly true to say that there is a 93% probability they are male, and a 7% probability they are female. If a rhomboid fossa is not observed then there is a 43% probability they are male and a 57% probability they are female. This makes possession of a rhomboid fossa a good indicator that skeletal remains came from a male skeleton, however, absence is a poor indicator for female skeletalized remains.

The conditional probabilities $\Pr(S_j \mid R_i)$ (Table 9.3) are not the same as $\Pr(R_i \mid S_j)$ (Table 9.4). For example, the 67% probability a male has a rhomboid fossa is *not* the same at all as the 93% probability an individual possessing a rhomboid fossa is male. The two different conditional probabilities make completely different statements about the data. Confusing the two is to commit the interpretational error of the transposed conditional, but is very easily done when describing these types of probabilities in words.

9.2 Bayes' theorem

In Section 3.1.4 we found that the probability of throwing a fair six-sided dice and it giving a score which was odd, event A, and greater than three, event B, could be calculated by the multiplication of $\Pr(A)$ and $\Pr(B|A)$.

The probability of event A, throwing an odd number, was $\Pr(A) = 1/2$, and the probability of throwing a number greater than three given the number was odd was $\Pr(B|A) = 1/3$. The probability for the joint event from these two dependent events was $\Pr(A, B) = 1/2 \times 1/3 = 1/6$. This is an illustration of Equation 2 which is termed the *third law of probability for dependent events*, and is simply $\Pr(A, B) = \Pr(A) \times \Pr(B|A)$.

What if we now reverse the order in which we do this calculation? The probability of rolling a score greater than three is $1/2$, as there are three possible scores greater than three from six possible scores, so now $\Pr(B) = 1/2$. If we have already rolled a score greater than three we are left with $x = \{4, 5, 6\}$ from which to roll an odd number. The probability of rolling an odd number given a number greater than three has already been rolled is now $Pr(A|B) = 1/3$ because the only score from x which is odd is 5. Multiplying these together we can say that $Pr(A, B) = Pr(B) \times Pr(A|B)$, or $1/2 \times 1/3 = 1/6$.

As $Pr(A, B)$ must equal $Pr(A, B)$ then:

$$Pr(A) \times Pr(B|A) = Pr(B) \times Pr(A|B)$$

or, rearranging by dividing through by $Pr(A)$:

$$Pr(B|A) = \frac{Pr(B) \times Pr(A|B)}{Pr(A)}$$

This is called Bayes' theorem, and simply relates unconditional probabilities to conditional probabilities.

Bayes' theorem can be used to make calculations for probabilities such as those found in Tables 9.3 and 9.4 through the unconditional probabilities found in Table 9.2. Using a change in notation, E to indicate evidence, and H to indicate hypothesis, Bayes' theorem can be rewritten:

$$Pr(H \mid E) = \frac{Pr(E \mid H) \times Pr(H)}{Pr(E)} \tag{22}$$

Equation 22 may be written more specifically for the example for the rhomboid fossa data above:

$$Pr(S_j \mid R_i) = \frac{Pr(R_i \mid S_j) \times Pr(S_j)}{Pr(R_i)} \tag{23}$$

Therefore, were one to examine a skeleton and find no rhomboid fossa one could calculate the probability of the sex being female by substitution into Equation 22, that is, given the observation of no rhomboid fossa we want the probability of sex female $(S_f \mid R_a)$ which is:

$$Pr(S_f \mid R_a) = \frac{Pr(R_a \mid S_f) \times Pr(S_f)}{Pr(R_a)}$$

The unconditional probabilities for sex are taken from the right-hand column of Table 9.2 are $Pr(S_f) = 0.33$, and for the absence of a rhomboid fossa from the bottom row of Table 9.2 $Pr(R_a) = 0.52$. From Table 9.4 the conditional probability for absence of a rhomboid fossa given sex is female is $Pr(R_a \mid S_f) = 0.89$; so:

$$Pr(S_f \mid R_a) = \frac{0.89 \times 0.33}{0.52}$$
$$= \frac{0.2937}{0.52}$$
$$\approx 0.57$$

or a 57% probability of a skeleton without a rhomboid fossa being from a female, which is exactly what we knew from the bottom right cell of Table 9.4.

Suppose that a rhomboid fossa were observed on the skeleton, what would be the probability that that skeleton were from a man? Rewriting Equation 23 for sex male and the presence of a rhomboid fossa we have:

$$Pr(S_m \mid R_p) = \frac{Pr(R_p \mid S_m) \times Pr(S_m)}{Pr(R_p)} \tag{24}$$

From the top right cell of Table 9.3 the probability of observing the presence of a rhomboid fossa given that the sex of the skeleton is male is $Pr(R_p|S_m) = 0.67$. From the right-hand column of Table 9.2 the probability of being male is $Pr(S_m) = 0.67$, and from the bottom row of Table 9.2 the probability of possessing a rhomboid fossa is $Pr(R_p) = 0.48$. Substituting these values into the equation above:

$$Pr(S_m \mid R_p) = \frac{0.67 \times 0.67}{0.48}$$
$$= \frac{0.4489}{0.48}$$
$$\approx 0.93$$

a probability confirmed by inspection of the top right cell for Table 9.4.

A useful variant on Equation 23 is to take the denominator $Pr(R_i)$ and expand it. From the bottom row of Table 9.2 the probability of $Pr(R_p)$ is 0.48. Using the *second law of probability* we know that this is equal to the sum of seeing the presence of a rhomboid fossa from males, and females. From the left farthest column of Table 9.2 we see this is $0.45 + 0.03 = 0.48$. What we can say then is:

$$Pr(R_p) = Pr(R_p, S_m) + Pr(R_p, S_f)$$

and from the *third law of probability for dependent events* we know:

$$Pr(R_p, S_m) = Pr(R_p|S_m) Pr(S_m)$$
$$Pr(R_p, S_f) = Pr(R_p|S_f) Pr(S_f)$$

so that $Pr(R_p) = [Pr(R_p|S_m) Pr(S_m)] + [Pr(R_p|S_f) Pr(S_f)]$. This means that Equation 24 can be rewritten:

$$Pr(S_m \mid R_p) = \frac{Pr(R_p \mid S_m) \times Pr(S_m)}{[Pr(R_p|S_m) Pr(S_m)] + [Pr(R_p|S_f) Pr(S_f)]} \tag{25}$$

From the top left cell of Table 9.3 $Pr(R_p|S_m) = 0.67$, from the bottom left cell $Pr(R_p|S_f) = 0.11$. From the right farthest column of Table 9.2 $Pr(S_m) = 0.67$, and,

$Pr(S_f) = 0.33$. Substituting these values into into the Equation 25 above:

$$Pr(S_m \mid R_p) = \frac{0.67 \times 0.67}{(0.67 \times 0.67) + (0.11 \times 0.33)}$$

$$= \frac{0.4489}{0.4852}$$

$$\approx 0.93$$

which is the expected probability from the top left cell in Table 9.4 for the probability that an individual was a man given the observation of a rhomboid fossa.

The probability of the sex of a skeleton given the presence or absence of a rhomboid fossa is called a *posterior probability*. At this point it must be wondered why one should go to the trouble of using Bayes' theorem to calculate the posterior probability for sex given the presence or absence of a rhomboid fossa when the posterior probabilities could just as well be looked up in Table 9.4. The reason is the unconditional probabilities $Pr(S_m)$ and $Pr(S_f)$ are called *prior probabilities* and are the probability of the sex of a skeleton before any information about the rhomboid fossa is taken into account. The prior probabilities used here which are dependent on the sample of skeletons to which we have had access, and are not prior probabilities from the number of males and females in a living population. From survey data we know the population is approximately 48% male and 52% female, not 67% male and 33% female as in the skeletal sample. So, were one inspecting a skeleton from an unknown source, rather than the sample, then it would be reasonable for $Pr(S_m) = 0.48$ and $Pr(S_f) = 0.52$. Carrying this out on the example above for the observation of a rhomboid fossa on a skeleton of unknown sex, then:

$$Pr(S_m \mid R_p) = \frac{0.67 \times 0.48}{(0.11 \times 0.52) + (0.67 \times 0.48)}$$

$$= \frac{0.3216}{0.0572 + 0.3216}$$

$$= 0.85$$

or an 85% probability that a skeleton with a rhomboid fossa is male, rather than the 93% probability suggested from when a prior probability from the data is used.

This is not the end of the process for a Bayesian type analysis. If there were some other sex indicator which was unrelated to the rhomboid fossa, then this could be used as an independent measure of sex. One way in which this could take form is to use the posterior probability of sex given the observation of the rhomboid fossa as the prior probability in another similar analysis. In this way pieces of independent evidence as to the sex of an unknown skeleton can be combined to give a probability for sex given all the indicators.

Bayes' theorem presents a flexible framework for the evaluation of probabilities, and one in which different and more realistic scenarios can be tried out using different prior information. The use of a Bayesian approach has been criticized for its use of prior information on the grounds that the investigator is 'just making it up', however, as we have seen from the example above, the substitution of survey priors for sample priors makes the attribution of a prior probability more reasonable. The use of a Bayesian approach allows us not only to use different assumptions about the data, but also forces us to examine these assumptions in some detail. More traditional approaches also make assumptions about the data, but these are not often as explicit as in the Bayesian approach.

9.3 The value of evidence

Illustrated above was a Bayesian approach to the estimation of sex by the observation of a skeletal feature. Central to the estimation process was the selection of a prior probability for sex. It is possible to select any reasonable, or even unreasonable, prior probability for any given analysis, and as long as the prior is a probability, and the conditioning is appropriate, then from a mathematical point of view the analysis itself is valid. The prior information in the example of the observation of a rhomboid fossa applied to an unknown skeleton from a population for which the male/female ratio is known is entirely reasonable.

Rather than thinking about male/female let us now think about the propositions of guilt or innocence of a suspect given some form of evidence.

As might be imagined, the selection of a prior would be problematic as the level of selection would be at issue. If, for example, a crime were committed in a town such as Rochdale with, according to the 2001 Census, 205 357 people, which in itself is in England with 49 138 991 people, is the prior probability of guilt for an individual 1/205 357 or 1/49 138 991?

Realistically such questions are impossible to answer, and not really a question with which the forensic scientist should be too concerned. Operationally the forensic scientist only sees a small amount of the evidence and is not in the same position as a jury in a criminal trial to make assessments of prior probabilities for the propositions of guilt or innocence. Also, it is not the role of the forensic scientists to give probabilities of guilt or innocence; their function is to comment solely on the evidence presented to them.

A way in which statisticians have overcome this problem is to derive a measure of the importance of the evidence. This is exactly the same measure of evidential value discussed in Section 8.3, but given here is a more mathematical treatment of the underlying rationale.

The first thing to consider are the odds of guilt. Odds are defined for an event w as:

$$\text{odds} = \frac{\text{probability of } w \text{ occurring}}{\text{probability of } w \text{ not occurring}}$$

An individual can only be truly guilty (G), or not guilty $(\overline{G})$[¶], can be written:

$$\text{odds}(G) = \frac{\Pr(G)}{\Pr(\overline{G})}$$

Conditioning on the evidence E:

$$\text{odds}(G \mid E) = \frac{\Pr(G \mid E)}{\Pr(\overline{G} \mid E)}.$$

Also, from Equation 25:

$$\Pr(G \mid E) = \frac{\Pr(E \mid G) \times \Pr(G)}{[\Pr(E \mid G) \times \Pr(G)] + [\Pr(E \mid \overline{G}) \times \Pr(\overline{G})]}$$

and:

$$\Pr(\overline{G} \mid E) = \frac{\Pr(E \mid \overline{G}) \times \Pr(\overline{G})}{[\Pr(E \mid \overline{G}) \times \Pr(\overline{G})] + [\Pr(E \mid G) \times \Pr(G)]}$$

Taking the ratio of the expressions above:

$$\frac{\Pr(G \mid E)}{Pr(\overline{G} \mid E)} = \frac{\dfrac{\Pr(E \mid G) \times \Pr(G)}{[\Pr(E \mid G) \times \Pr(G)] + [\Pr(E \mid \overline{G}) \times \Pr(\overline{G})]}}{\dfrac{\Pr(E \mid \overline{G}) \times \Pr(\overline{G})}{[\Pr(E \mid \overline{G}) \times \Pr(\overline{G})] + [\Pr(E \mid G) \times \Pr(G)]}}$$

$$= \frac{\Pr(E \mid G) \times \Pr(G) \times \{[\Pr(E \mid G) \times \Pr(G)] + [\Pr(E \mid \overline{G}) \times \Pr(\overline{G})]\}}{\Pr(E \mid \overline{G}) \times \Pr(\overline{G}) \times \{[\Pr(E \mid G) \times \Pr(G)] + [\Pr(E \mid \overline{G}) \times \Pr(\overline{G})]\}}$$

$$= \frac{\Pr(E \mid G) \times \Pr(G)}{\Pr(E \mid \overline{G}) \times \Pr(\overline{G})}$$

$$= \frac{\Pr(E \mid G)}{\Pr(E \mid \overline{G})} \times \frac{\Pr(G)}{\Pr(\overline{G})} \qquad\qquad (26)$$

The various components of Equation 26 are listed below:

$$\underbrace{\frac{\Pr(G \mid E)}{\Pr(\overline{G} \mid E)}}_{\text{Posterior odds}} = \underbrace{\frac{\Pr(E \mid G)}{\Pr(E \mid \overline{G})}}_{\text{Likelihood ratio}} \times \underbrace{\frac{\Pr(G)}{\Pr(\overline{G})}}_{\text{Prior odds}}$$

The prior odds and the posterior odds of guilt are for the consideration of the court in criminal cases, the scientist being in no position to evaluate either. The only feature of Equation 26 which is directly dependent on the evidence and the propositions to which that evidence lends support, but is not influenced by the prior odds, is the

[¶]The converse of guilty is written here as $\overline{G}$ where the bar above the G means not.

likelihood ratio, which is

$$LR = \frac{\Pr(E \mid G)}{\Pr(E \mid \overline{G})} \tag{27}$$

and exactly the measure of evidential value discussed in Section 8.3.

Review questions

1. As part of their work on the frequency and type of bone lesions caused by gun-shot wounds in skeletal material de la Grandmaison *et al.* (2001 reproduced with permission) give the following survey as part of their findings.

	homicide	suicide
skull	33	34
spine	16	1
torso	29	13
limbs	12	1

The entries in the table are the number of individual corpses with the known cause of firearm-inflicted-wounding in each part of their anatomy. Assume one wound was inflicted on each individual.

(a) What is the probability that someone from the sample was the victim of a homicide?

(b) What is the probability of observing an individual from the sample who has committed suicide by shooting themselves in the torso?

(c) What is the probability that someone who has been murdered has spinal gunshot wound?

(d) What is the probability that someone who has a spinal gunshot wound has been murdered?

(e) What is the probability that someone from the sample committed suicide if a gunshot wound were inflicted in their left leg?

(f) What is the probability that someone from the sample who has a gunshot wound to the left leg committed suicide? Assume each limb to be equally likely to be injured in any suicide attempt.

2. Suppose there are about 1500 suicides and 800 homicides in the UK each year, and that if a body is found in the UK with gunshot wounds, and the only explanations are suicide or homicide. Use the data from Question 1 from de la Grandmaison *et al.*

(2001) to answer the following:

(a) If a body is found with gunshot wounds to the left leg what is the probability the wounds are the result of homicide?
(b) If a body is found with gunshot wounds to the head what is the probability that the wounds are the result of homicide?
(c) If a body has been found in which the individual is known to have committed suicide, what is the probability that the body has a gunshot wound to the torso?

10 Relevance and the formulation of propositions

Thus far we have discussed evidence in the face of two propositions: that the suspect is guilty, and the suspect is innocent. We have taken it for granted that the evidence in the examples we have examined somehow points to one or the other of these two extremes. Obviously these two propositions are gross simplifications to allow for the clear explanation of the statistical principles which are the proper subject of this book, but it has been suggested (Kind, 1994) that the use of propositions which refer directly to 'guilt' or 'innocence' are the province of the court, and not the forensic scientist. However, in casework proposition formulation is a crucial element of evidence evaluation as data only become, and a evidence when set against the propositional framework to which those data are supposed to be relevant. In fact, in many cases, the mathematical computations are trivial: it is the formulation of the set of propositions in which the observations are to be evaluated which is the most challenging stage of the process process which itself can have a profound effect on the calculation of evidential value (Meester and Sjerps, 2004).

But what property of any particular set of observations is it which causes an individual to have belief that events in the world has a given form over any other form? The answer must have something to do with an association at some level, either by the constant conjugation of similar observations with similar states, or the formulation of some logical relationship between those observations and world states. This property has been termed *relevance*.

10.1 Relevance

The general term used in United Kingdom jurisdictions for the property linking observation to a legal state is relevance. Roberts and Zuckerman (2004) put it this way: 'x is relevant to y for our purposes if x contributes towards proving or disproving y'. This definition is a little circular and not overly helpful, but is as specific as one

Introduction to Statistics for Forensic Scientists　David Lucy
© 2005 John Wiley & Sons, Ltd.

can be without narrowing the definition so much that it fails to cover all statements considered relevant.

In United Kingdom jurisdictions there is no lower limit to how much any piece of evidence should bear on the legal issue under consideration. Evidence is either relevant, or not relevant (Roberts and Zuckerman, 2004). This means that, in principle at least, any evidence, provided it fulfils the criteria above, would be counted as relevant. Of course, in practice, there are non-evidential constraints on courts such as time and resource limits which may be significant in a court's decision as to what evidence might be considered relevant. Other constraints might be those of admissibility and the notion of a fair trial where evidence, no matter how relevant and powerfully indicative in a case, if illegally collected, would not be brought before the court.

The problem is that although the concept of relevance exists, both in a legal sense and a common sense, it is difficult to think of it as a single conceptual entity. Roberts and Zuckerman (2004) discuss the work of Hohfeld who thought about a division of evidence into *constitutive facts* and *evidential facts*. Constitutive facts are what, for the sake of simplicity, we have been structuring our hypotheses around, the fact of guilt or innocence in law, or in lawyers' parlance the *ultimate issue*. These might be that some offender actually did break into a house by means of forcing the door with a crowbar. In this case the offender would be guilty of the offence of breaking and entering.

Evidential facts are those material facts which by some leap of inference lead to a constitutive fact. Such a fact may be that a suspect owns a crowbar, and a genetic profile from bloodstain from a crimescene where a house has been broken into matches the profile of the suspect. In this case it is an evidential fact that the suspect owns a crowbar, and a further evidential fact that a profile matching that of the suspect has been found at a crimescene. These when considered together may lead, by an inferential leap, to the constitutive fact that the suspect had been guilty of breaking and entering. The inferential leap is critical, in that the possession of a crowbar does not by necessity indicate that the suspect had used it to gain access to the house in question, nor does the genetic profile lead with any logical certainty to the conclusion that the suspect has been guilty of house breaking.

10.2 Hierarchy of propositions

A conceptually similar scheme of more relevance to forensic science was outlined by Cook *et al.* (1998). Here any proposition is envisaged as belonging in a category within a hierarchy of propositions. The categories, in hierarchical order, are source, activity and offence. The source level would fit into Hohfeld's evidential fact, although it is an elaboration of Hohfeld's classification. Source level propositions are those which are at the level of much day-to-day forensic science, particularly processes such as comparison to assess whether or not some trace at a crimescene could have been left by some suspect. Propositions addressed at the level of 'is the DNA profile from the suspect or not?', or, 'is this glass likely to have come from this bottle or not?' are all the source level.

The activity level is considered above the source level in the hierarchy of propositions, in that in many cases it might be easier directly to relate a suspect's actions to criminal activity than it would source level propositions. As with the source level the activity level can be related directly to Hohfeld's evidential fact type. Activity level propositions require more than the execution of a matching exercise. To evaluate propositions at this level it is necessary to consider information other than direct observational data. In the example above such questions would be 'was the bloodstain on the broken door?', if so, 'is this the sort of bloodstain which might be expected on a forced door?'. If the bloodstain were from a razor in the bathroom then an activity level proposition may not be sustained.

The final level is the offence level, and is loosely equivalent to Hohfeld's constitutive fact, and is the level at which a jury could be expected to consider the case.

In reality the categories described by Cook *et al.* (1998) are not absolute. There is some overlap between them. For example, a suspect may well open a door by means of a crowbar, but if it is their own door then no crime has been committed. Evaluation at the source and activity level of propositions would look very similar to a criminal case of breaking and entering, but at the offence level there would be no case to answer.

The activity level can be viewed by forensic scientists as the most productive level in the hierarchy as they force evidence to be examined which might not be considered were only the source level to be in question. As a development of their ideas Evett *et al.* (2000a) consider the role of explanation in evidence evaluation, and the distinctions between explanations and propositions. In short, an explanation can be any set of reasons which explain the world state of the evidence. Propositions must come in pairs and have some tightly knitted logical interrelation with the circumstances of the case. An explanation for a DNA profile matching that of a suspect in the breaking and entering case above could be that an individual with the same profile was the offender. If this were the case then the probability that the two profiles would exactly match given the suspect were the offender would be 1, and the probability the two profiles would match given that the offender had the same profile as the suspect would also be 1, giving a non-informative likelihood ratio of 1. However, in the transformation to a proposition network the implications for the explanation in respect of the case would have to be taken into account, so the propositions might be that the probability of an exact match given that the suspect was the true source of the DNA profile might again be 1. However, the defence case may be one of the probability of an exact match given that someone with the same DNA profile was the true source of the crimescene profile, and who was not the suspect. This probability would not necessarily be 1. The difference is that the defence proposition is formulated taking into account the circumstances of the case and the prosecution proposition with the observation that the offender would also have to be someone other than the suspect were the defence proposition true.

10.3 Likelihood ratios and relevance

The measure of likelihood ratio seems an obvious candidate to supplant more legal notions of relevance. Broadly, the closer a likelihood ratio is to 1 then the less relevant the evidence. Unfortunately not all evidence can be evaluated by a likelihood ratio and, as seen above, proposition formulation is very much informed by commonsensical, and legal, ideas about relevance. This means that to calculate a likelihood ratio requires some framework of propositions, which in its turn require some ideas about the relevance of the evidence. Thus it is difficult to conceive of a likelihood ratio as a neutral measure of the relevance of evidence without invoking some form of tautology.

Researchers have thought about a more formal approach to including a measure of relevance into likelihood ratio calculations. Stoney (1991) considered a case where it was uncertain whether a piece of evidence recovered from the scene of a crime had in fact been left by the offender. The illustration below is a simplified version of Evett's (1993) generalization of this notion of relevance to a situation where it is uncertain whether or not evidence of some categorical nature is observed at a crimescene as a result of the offender's activity.

A general form for such evidence is:

$$LR = \frac{Pr(E \mid H_p)}{Pr(E \mid H_d)} \tag{28}$$

where E is the evidence that there is a match between some property of the suspect and crimescene which occurs with frequency f in the appropriate population. Let H_p be the activity level proposition that the suspect undertook some actions which would have resulted in the transfer of the evidence, and H_d is activity level proposition that someone other than the suspect undertook some actions which resulted in transfer of the evidence. Let B denote the proposition that the evidential material was connected with the offence, and $\overline{B}$ will represent the proposition that the material was not connected with the offence. Using the *second law of probability*, Equation 28 can be rewritten:

$$LR = \frac{Pr(E, B \mid H_p) + Pr(E, \overline{B} \mid H_p)}{Pr(E, B \mid H_d) + Pr(E, \overline{B} \mid H_d)} \tag{29}$$

From the *third law of probability for dependent events* we know $Pr(A, B \mid H) = Pr(A \mid B, H) Pr(B \mid H)$, therefore Equation 29 can also be rewritten:

$$LR = \frac{\Pr(E \mid B, H_p)\Pr(B \mid H_p) + \Pr(E \mid \overline{B}, H_p)\Pr(\overline{B} \mid H_p)}{\Pr(E \mid B, H_d)\Pr(B \mid H_d) + \Pr(E \mid \overline{B}, H_d)\Pr(\overline{B} \mid H_d)}$$

Because our knowledge of the suspect's activities does not affect our belief in whether the evidence was connected with the offence B is independent of H:

$$LR = \frac{\Pr(E \mid B, H_p)\Pr(B) + \Pr(E \mid \overline{B}, H_p)\Pr(\overline{B})}{\Pr(E \mid B, H_d)\Pr(B) + \Pr(E \mid \overline{B}, H_d)\Pr(\overline{B})} \tag{30}$$

If we denote r as the probability that the evidence is connected with the offence that is ρ is a relevance term, then $\Pr(B)$ is equal to r, so $\Pr(\overline{B})$ will equal $1 - r$ as these are complementary propositions, that is, the evidence was connected with the offence, or it was not. If the evidence was connected with the offence, and the suspect undertook actions which would result in the transfer of the evidence, then the evidence is inevitable, or $\Pr(E|B, H_p) = 1$. If the evidential material was not connected with the offence, and just happens to be there by some other means, the evidence does not depend on the suspect's activities, so $\Pr(E \mid \overline{B}, H_p) = \Pr(E \mid \overline{B}) = \Pr(E) = f$. If the suspect did not undertake any activities which would have resulted in the evidence, but the material was connected with the offence then $\Pr(E \mid B, H_d) = \Pr(E \mid B) = \Pr(E) = f$. If the evidence was not connected with the offence, and the suspect's activities did not result in the transfer of the evidential material, then again the evidence was from some other source, so $\Pr(E \mid \overline{B}, H_d) = \Pr(E) = f$. Substituting these values into Equation 30 we have:

$$LR = \frac{1 \times r + f \times (1 - r)}{f \times r + f \times (1 - r)}$$

$$= \frac{r + f(1 - r)}{rf + f(1 - r)}$$

$$= \frac{r + f(1 - r)}{rf + f - rf}$$

$$= \frac{r + f(1 - r)}{f}$$

This sort of approach to the uncertainty in the source of evidence have been generalized to where evidence may have been transferred from the crimescene to a suspect, and where there may be two traces from the crimescene and more than one suspect (Evett, 1993; Stoney, 1994).

This idea of relevance as a probabilistic function relating material found at a crimescene, and on a suspect, runs counter to the more binary legal idea of relevance, and is intuitively more realistic than declaring evidence 'relevant' or 'not relevant' to the offence in question. However, finding suitable values for r will pose many problems for those wishing to include a relevance term in their calculations.

10.4 The logic of relevance

We have seen that the answers given by forensic scientists to forensic data should be framed in terms of a series of propositions about some state of the world. This state should have some underlying empirical relationship to the offence in question. However, an empirical relationship is not a logical relationship. In our example the forensic evidence would point directly at a source level. The propositions from the forensic scientist would at this point be about the source of the DNA profile, and whether it belonged to the suspect, or some other unknown person. The crowbar belonging to the suspect could also be treated similarly to produce some evaluation of the source of the crowbar and marks made upon the door of the property which was broken into. By consideration of the background circumstances it would be possible to extend the argument to making a statement about the suspect having levered open the door. However, this in itself does not logically entail the constitutive fact that the suspect was guilty of breaking and entering. It would not even sustain the offence of criminal damage even if it were established that the door had been forced by the suspect, as the suspect's purpose for levering the door open would have to be considered. As stated earlier the relationship between activity and offence is not one which is usually open to direct inference from the evidential facts. The higher level *ultimate* issue has to be decided by some other means.

Roberts and Zuckerman (2004) give three ways in which this is done in English law. The first is that there may be a coincidence between the language in which the constitutive fact is stated and a common understanding of that fact. In the example above, were no extenuating circumstances known as to why the suspect should damage the door then the activity of forcing the door open would establish the constitutive fact of criminal damage. Commonality of meaning, although a simple means of turning activity level propositions into offence level propositions, carries with it the problem that language changes in meaning and is somewhat fuzzy in its usage. Also this might not necessarily apply to the constitutive fact of breaking and entering unless – and this brings us to the second method by which English law can relate activity to offence, which is to define breaking and entering as entering in any form. This might include the tip of an implement. So were the door forced, then at least the tip of the crowbar would enter the premises, and the constitutive fact might be established by definition. This almost goes too far the other way in that for every offence the minute details of what constitutes that offence would have to be defined in some manner, and would-be offenders armed with knowledge of the law could still undertake acts which, although deeply anti-social and offensive, would nevertheless avoid by the slimmest of margins being a criminal offence. English law has very few instances where the evidential fact at the activity level would lead directly to a constitutive fact. The statutary offence of rape comes quite close to this situation, and is very tightly defined in English law, although the suspect must be shown to have intended 'to commit intercourse', but as with most questions of intent, the suspect's state of mind has to be inferred from their activities[†].

The third mechanism which can link evidential facts and constitutive facts, and the one preferred in the English criminal law, is the commonsense judgement of the jury. In the fictitious case above, the jury might decide that the evidence supported a case for the constitutive fact that the suspect was guilty of breaking and entering based upon their own reasoning about the activity of door forcing, that is, 'why force the door if entry was not the intention?'. On the other hand, given all the evidence, the jury may not even think that the constitutive fact of criminal damage is sustained, despite the evidence of the activity level.

10.5 The formulation of propositions

To be of probative value forensic evidence must in some way be able to relate evidential facts to constitutive facts. From the argument above, except in the case where constitutive facts can be narrowly framed, and in some senses set equal to propositions made at the activity level, this is simply not possible in any direct manner.

So what is possible? The constitutive fact 'the suspect committed an offence of breaking and entering' must imply that there was somewhere to break and enter, and that someone had broken and entered. Unfortunately it does not imply activity level statements such as 'forced the door with a crowbar', and it certainly does not imply source level statements such as 'the DNA profile from a bloodstain found at the crimescene matches the profile of the suspect'. All we do by using evidential facts to support constitutive claims is to offer up a possibility, or possibilities, which may be one or a few selected from an unknown number of alternative possibilities, unless the connection is so obvious as might be the case where there is a first-hand eyewitness to all the activities said to comprise the offence.

A fruitful approach dependent on the constitutive fact in question, may be to approach the formulation of propositions from the point of view of those whose task it is to assess the evidential facts in relation to the constitutive facts. In English criminal law this may be the jury. The forensic scientist might seek to formulate their hypotheses by using their shared cultural notions of the putative constitutive fact in the context of the activity and source level evidential facts in a way similar to that described by Collingwood (1946), where all facts are thought of as being a logical consequence of a sensible viewpoint. When the question is 'what sort of viewpoint considers these facts as sensible?', discover the viewpoint and the question is to some extent solved. Collingwood's work is reflected in more modern discourses on narratives, and the view that facts are given coherence by some sequence of temporal and causative relationships deduced from everyday experience

---

[†] Schafer *pers. comm.*

(Edmond, 1999; Junker, 1998). This work has been extended to a more formal structure by Prakken (2004).

Another source of propositions might be those suggested by other parts of the court, such as those in an advocacy role. Here the forensic scientist might have less of a part to play in the evaluation of their evidence.

In practice, those responsible for selecting hypotheses will take into account what they know of the evidence in any case, the offence level propositions, what advocates on either side may say, and, most critically of all, what can be told from the material evidence. However, it is a process involving human judgement and human intellects, and not some wholly mechanical process. Common logic, and the investigation of structures such as narratives, can be useful for discounting propositions which may be incompatible with the data, or incoherent in some way, but do not act as a sure guide as to what propositions should be stated.

10.6 What kind of propositions can we not evaluate?

The mathematical principles of evidence evaluation are in a sense blind, in that they are logically the same as long as their basic tenets are adhered to irrespective of the propositions under evaluation, and the data used in that evaluation. We can, in principle, evaluate propositions for which suitable data exist for any set of propositions, but should we? Are there classes of propositions which should not be evaluated, or, at least if they are, those evaluations should not be used as evidence in formal proceedings.

When presented with matching characteristics where those characteristics may be from a shoe, garment, weapon, or any of the other transferred materials found at crimescenes and in the possession of suspects, a suitable database may be described. If a database can be specified then statistical evaluation of the evidence is a rational thing to do. Similarly with evidence which is of numerical form, such as glass compositional measurements, where examination of the evidence itself without a statistical approach is difficult, a statistical evaluation of that evidence may be the only way of establishing any form of probative value for the data.

But what about areas such as eyewitness statements? An eyewitness statement may point unambiguously to a suspect, and give evidence at the activity, or even offence levels of proposition. The uncertainties here are associated with the veracity of the witness, or the accuracy of the witness, but not the evidence itself. Can we place a numerical probability on eyewitness statements? Legal procedures exist to make some gross inferences about whether an eyewitness's abilities are consistent with their statement, and whether the witness is suitable in other respects, such as not being the suspect's spouse in certain offence categories, and other types of admissibility rule (Redmayne, 2001). However, is it possible to place some other more direct value on the strength of the eyewitness's evidence?

It would be possible to perform a 'lie detector' experiment on the witness, and evaluate the evidence from the resultant data, or to see how often the witness had told falsehoods under similar circumstances in the past. Unfortunately these experiments, in the unlikely event that they would give a good indication of the witness's state of mind, would only tell us whether the witness was telling a conscious untruth, and would not give any indication of whether the witness was simply mistaken. The point is that there is nothing quantitatively measurable about an eyewitness which can have any relevance to the veracity of their testimony besides those rules already established by the criminal courts.

The same is true for evidence which is on a relative scale. If a suspect is described as being 'tall', what is the meaning of 'tall'? In this case it would be possible to perform an experiment whereby the witness observed individuals described as tall, and the parameters used from the sample to define a numerical equivalent of tall, but the description of tall by itself without the data from the experiment could not be evaluated.

Although marks from footwear can be reliably used to give the type of footwear used by an offender, and that the type of footwear would usually be easy to evaluate as evidence from knowledge of the frequencies of the observed footwear, what about further acquired features of that footwear? Footmark examiners can match acquired features on footwear from a mark to a print taken from a suspect shoe and, if the features match, these can serve as further evidence that the shoe which made the mark at the crimescene was that from the suspect observed by the examiner. Can acquired marks on footwear be regarded as unique features identifying the particular shoe, and that shoe only? In some circumstances yes, if, for instance, someone has branded the sole of the shoe with their name, then this might be seen as unique, although there is absolutely no logical reason to believe that some shoe, somewhere, does not have the same mark upon it. Wear and tear characteristics will be related to the shoe type, that is, some shoes will wear in particular ways, the wearer's gait, and the purpose to which the shoe is put. These sorts of acquired traits may, or may not, further identify the particular shoe.

It would be possible to conduct a survey of shoes of a given type, and from that estimate the frequency of the acquired characteristics in question. However, at the time of writing this is not a realistic proposition due to the levels of work involved. Also, the acquired characteristics which footwear examiners observe are dynamic in that they are subject to change, and although mathematical modelling of these changes would be possible, any model concieved of in the near future would be unlikely to exceed the performance of an expert examiner.

This should also be true of all evidence types which are fundamentally about the identification of classes of object. For instance, the evidential value for types of firearm, or motor vehicles, can usually be evaluated fairly easily. The further evidence of modification, either intentional, or as a result of use, used by experts in the particular field is not so straightforward. However, as acquired features always act further to individualize a piece of evidence, the exact value of the type of evidence can be seen as a lower bound to any further information which any such acquired features may add. So the evidence from the 'match' of characteristics seen in association with a crimescene and evidence associated with a suspect can have two components, an easily evaluated numerical value given by the type and relevant databases which forms a lower bound to the value of this piece of evidence, and a component given by the non-numeric evaluation of the expert examiner.

A form of evidence which it might be reasonably straightforward to evaluate from a statistical point of view, but which would present problems from a legal perspective, would be circumstantial evidence based upon a suspect's social characteristics. For instance, were a street robbery to be committed, and a suspect detained, and the suspect happened to be drug dependent, then is the fact that the suspect is drug dependent of any probative value?

It would not be straightforward, but not impossible, to estimate the probability of someone committing a street robbery were they drug dependent, and of someone committing street robbery were they not drug dependent. From a survey of the population a prior probability for drug dependency could be calculated, so the transposed probabilities may be calculated. However, this sort of evidence is purely circumstantial; it is not known whether the offender was drug dependent or not. If this were known, then the evidence could be treated in the same way as any other evidence of matching characteristics. All that is known is that the suspect is drug-dependent. This may give evidence of motive, but cannot be treated as a piece of evidence directly for the involvement of the suspect even were it to turn out that drug-dependent individuals are more likely than non-drug dependents to commit street robbery.

The whole area of circumstantial evidence is a very difficult one philosophically, but, in principle at least, some areas can be easily treated mathematically. Take, for instance, a piece of circumstantial evidence such as the observation of nine fires over a period of years in the residences of a suspect in an arson case, and no innocent explanation forthcoming. Establishing a probability of a member of the general public, who is not suspected of arson, experiencing nine fires at their residences is calculable, possibly from the records of insurance companies. Some estimate of the probability of an arsonist setting nine fires in their own residences can, in principle, from past cases of arson, be calculated. Therefore the evidence can be evaluated. But can this really be evidence in the same way as the observation of some characteristic shared between suspect and offender?

Certainly common sense suggests that an individual who has experienced nine fires when none might be expected might be suspected of arson on the basis of the observation, but does the evidence point to arson, misfortune or undue carelessness? Has a crime been committed at all? In the case where a door has been forced and a residence broken into it has been established that a crime has been committed before any evidential observations have been made. The same may not be true in the arson case. Unless there is other evidence such as the observation of fire setting materials by a fire examiner at the scenes of the fires, the role of the evidential nature of the record of fires has to be questioned. Is it evidence that the criminal offence of arson has been undertaken, or is it evidence that a specific individual has been responsible for that criminal offence? The evaluation of an observation of this sort of circumstantial evidence revolves around which propositions are under evaluation, and whether they relevant to the constitutive fact of arson.

This sort of evidence came forward in the trial of Dr Harold Shipman who, it was found, had been murdering elderly ladies at his practice in Hyde, Greater Manchester, England. Suspicion fell upon him in 1998 from members of the undertaking profession, who observed unusually high numbers of deaths from his practice, and clinical practitioners in adjoining practices who were obliged to countersign the death certificates he issued. Shipman was arrested in July 1998 when the daughter of one of his victims reported to police that her mother's Will was a forgery made by Shipman.

Shipman was convicted of the murder of 15 of his patients by the administration of diamorphine. Most of the physical evidence revolved around the detection of the metabolic products of morphine in the tissue of the patients for whom morphine had not been prescribed. Other evidence included the recovery of surgery records which had been altered, and eyewitness testimony to his behaviour at the time of his victims' deaths. The evidence of the numbers of patients who died in his care was only a peripheral feature of the case against Shipman, one which took on greater significance in post-conviction reviews surrounding the circumstances of the case (Baker, 2001). It is estimated that throughout his career Shipman murdered in excess of 160 individuals. One must wonder whether, were the numbers of deaths the only evidence, a criminal conviction could have been substantiated against Shipman.

11 Evaluation of evidence in practice

The process of the evaluation of evidence, particularly scientific evidence, can be statistically based. However, from Chapter 10 it is clear that statistical considerations need to be thought about in a context of, and body of theory which is not provided by statistical science. The statistical matters are, in some senses, only the tools by which evidence can be measured. There are other non-statistical, but crucial, elements in the evaluation of evidence which come about as a consequence of evidence evaluation being a very practical application of quantitative methods to law.

11.1 Which database to use

Underlying the use of a statistical measure of evidential value is the expectation that the required probabilities are derived from a database which is appropriate. In this Section we shall discuss some of the factors which are important in database selection, and later see how to avoid some of the pitfalls of interpretation such as the defendants database fallacy.

Type and geographic factors

Consider a crime to have been committed, and a shoemark found at the scene of the offence. It is thought that the mark belonged to the offender. Let us imagine a suspect has been apprehended, and has a pair of shoes which have been identified as being of the same type as the offender's. There are no acquired marks which could be used further to identify the shoe of the offender as distinguishable from the crimescene mark, nor the suspect's shoes. What sort of population does one need to establish the frequency of the shoes in question?

There are two considerations, the first is the type of shoe, the second is the geographical limit of the population under examination.

Introduction to Statistics for Forensic Scientists   David Lucy
© 2005 John Wiley & Sons, Ltd.

In the United Kingdom shoemarks from crimescenes tend to be of the 'training shoe' variety, although by no means always. So one figure which may be considered if the shoe is a training shoe is the frequency of the particular shoe amongst all training shoes. This would not be entirely correct as workboots, dress shoes and casual shoes have in the past been worn by individuals committing criminal acts. In fact a more correct population to examine would be one which comprised any footwear *fit for purpose* of committing the criminal act. This category might exclude divers boots, carpet slippers and shoes with stiletto heels, but might include Wellington boots and plimsolls. Were one only to include those shoes of a classification similar to the offender's shoe classification, for example training shoes, then the frequency would be severely overestimated, that overestimation being in the suspect's favour. This may, or may not, present a problem in the context of the case being made.

The geographical limit of the potential suspect population must also be thought about. Wetherby is a small town in North Yorkshire. North Yorkshire is an administrative area of England. Were the crime mentioned above to have been committed in Wetherby does one use the frequency of the particular shoe type in Wetherby, in North Yorkshire, the frequency of the shoe type in England, in the United Kingdom, or indeed the world? We must bear in mind what frequency we are trying to assess here. That frequency is the frequency of the particular shoe type in the population of potential suspects. It the offence were burglary then the investigator might think that the offender came from Wetherby, and that therefore the frequency required would be the frequency of the shoe type in that town. On the other hand there might be good reason to think that the offender was from somewhere else in North Yorkshire, and that a frequency for the whole of North Yorkshire might be the most suitable. In this instance it is a matter for the experience and expertise of the investigator to choose the geographical location of the potential suspect population.

What happens if it is thought the most suitable potential population of suspects was the population of Weatherby, but the only data available were for North Yorkshire, or England? All we are trying to do is estimate a frequency, if the frequency of the shoes in England is no different from Wetherby, then we have the correct frequency, and no more needs to be done. It is where there is good reason to suspect that a frequency may be different where one should be careful. For instance, if is it known that 30 000 pairs of the shoes above were made in the Orient, and imported to the United Kingdom, do we use the population of all fit for purpose shoes in the world, a very high number indeed, to estimate the frequency of the shoe in question in Wetherby? No, this would be incorrect as the shoes in question were not distributed uniformly throughout the world, they were all imported into the United Kingdom. If the shoes had been exported and sold in all parts of the world then it may be appropriate to estimate the frequency of the particular type of shoe from the whole world population of shoes.

As it is, if the shoe type were uniformly distributed throughout the United Kingdom, then it would be appropriate to estimate the frequency of the shoe type from all those fit for purpose shoes in the United Kingdom. However, if shoe type in question were more popular in North Yorkshire than in, say, Cardiff, then the frequency for North Yorkshire should be used. Needless to say that were the frequency for Wetherby different from the rest of North Yorkshire then the frequencies for Wetherby would have to be used.

DNA and database selection

Evett and Weir (1998) relate the case in 1991 of Mr Passino who was on trial for homicide in Vermont. There was a clear link formed by DNA evidence between Passino and the crime, but the defence argued that the DNA be ruled as inadmissible on the grounds that Passino's paternal grandparents were Italian, his maternal grandfather Native American, and his maternal grandmother half Native American and half French, and that there existed no databases of DNA from French-Native American-Italians.

Is it correct that the appropriate DNA database to use is that of the suspect to evaluate DNA evidence?

Aitken and Taroni (2004) point out that the direction of transfer of source material will affect the calculation of a suitable likelihood ratio (for a proof see Evett, 1984), however, each direction can ultimately be reduced to the other, so only the case where the direction is from the offender to the crimescene is considered here.

In the most general sense let us consider a genotype γ, and a sub-population ϕ. Let a crime be committed, and a genotype γ be recovered from the scene of the crime. If a suspect is apprehended and they have genotype γ, and happen to be from sub-population ϕ, then what is the value of the observation of γ taking into account the effect of ϕ?

If we take into account the suspect's membership of ϕ then there are three pieces of evidence. Let E_p be the observation that the suspect is a member of ϕ, E_s be the evidence that the suspect is of genotype γ, and E_c be the evidence that γ is observed from material recovered from the crimescene. We wish to evaluate this evidence within the framework of two opposing hypotheses, H_p is the source level hypothesis that the material from which γ was recovered came from the suspect, and H_d be the hypothesis that the material from which γ was recovered came from some source other than the suspect. So:

$$\mathbf{V} = \frac{\Pr(E \mid H_p)}{\Pr(E \mid H_d)}$$

$$= \frac{\Pr(E_p, E_s, E_c \mid H_p)}{\Pr(E_p, E_s, E_c \mid H_d)}$$

This can be rewritten:

$$= \frac{\Pr(E_p, E_s \mid E_c, H_p)}{\Pr(E_p, E_s \mid E_c, H_d)} \frac{\Pr(E_c \mid H_p)}{\Pr(E_c \mid H_d)}$$

where E_c, the evidence that γ is observed at the crimescene, will be independent of whether the material recovered from the crimescene came from the suspect, or some source other than the crimescene. The equation above can therefore be written:

$$= \frac{Pr(E_p, E_s \mid E_c, H_p)}{Pr(E_p, E_s \mid E_c, H_d)}$$

$$= \frac{Pr(E_p \mid E_c, H_p)}{Pr(E_p \mid E_c, H_d)} \frac{Pr(E_s \mid E_p, E_c, H_p)}{Pr(E_s \mid E_p, E_c, H_d)}$$

which if (H_d), the suspect was not the donor for the material from the crimescene of genotype γ, then both E_p and E_s will be independent of E_c, so the equation above can be stated:

$$= \frac{Pr(E_p \mid E_c, H_p)}{Pr(E_p \mid H_d)} \frac{Pr(E_s \mid E_p, E_c, H_p)}{Pr(E_s \mid E_p, H_d)} \tag{31}$$

The elements in the equation (above) are: $Pr(E_p \mid E_c, H_p)$, which is the probability the suspect came from the sub-population ϕ, where genotype γ was observed at the crimescene, and the suspect donated the material of genotype γ, this can be written $Pr(\gamma \mid \phi)$. $Pr(E_p \mid H_d)$ is the probability that the suspect is from sub-population ϕ given the suspect did not donate the material from which γ was observed. If the suspect did not donate the material from which γ was observed then this reduces to $Pr(\phi)$ which is the frequency of observing members of the sub-population ϕ in the population at large. $Pr(E_s \mid E_p, E_c, H_p)$ is the probability that the suspect is of genotype γ given the crimescene material is of genotype γ, the suspect is from sub-population ϕ and the suspect had donated that material. As the suspect has only one genotype to donate then this must be evaluated as 1. $Pr(E_s \mid E_p, H_d)$ is the probability that the suspect is of genotype γ given the suspect is from sub-population ϕ, and someone other than the suspect donated that material, which is the probability of observing γ given sub-population ϕ, or $Pr(\gamma \mid \phi)$.

Rewriting Equation 31 we have:

$$\mathbf{V} = \frac{Pr(\phi \mid \gamma)}{Pr(\phi) Pr(\gamma \mid \phi)}.$$

From Bayes' theorem (Equation 22):

$$Pr(\gamma) = \frac{Pr(\phi) Pr(\gamma \mid \phi)}{Pr(\phi \mid \gamma)}$$

so:

$$\mathbf{V} = \frac{1}{Pr(\gamma)}.$$

If we take the additional information that the suspect is from sub-population ϕ, we have exactly the same frequency had we used the frequency of γ in the wider population. Thus the effect of the suspect's membership of sub-population ϕ is irrelevant, and that the appropriate population from which find the frequency for γ is the wider population of potential suspects.

In summary, the essential point is that a suitable database will be from the wider population of what are known about the offender characteristics. That is, if it is thought the offender is from some specific geographical area, and the evidence, say some outer garment, which matches between suspect and crimescene, then the evidential value would be the observation of the matching outer garment amongst all fit for purpose garments in that specific geographical area. The population of fit for purpose outer garments can be constrained to some specific type of outer garment, such as overcoats, even if the constraint is not wholly justified, as this is a sub-section of total fit for purpose outer garments, and the approximation will favour the suspect. The issue of geographical area can also be relaxed if it is thought that the frequency of the matching article in a wider geographical area is no different from that of the specific area as the evidential value for the match will not change.

The same rule applies to immutable forms of evidence such as DNA. If a suspect is apprehended and the evidence is they have is a DNA match to some DNA recovered from a crimescene and no innocent explanation for its presence, then the appropriate database to examine for the frequency of the particular genotype is that of the wider population in the area, as nothing is known about the offender except that they have a DNA profile matching that of the suspect. More difficult cases where there may be contradictory evidence, such as a matching DNA profile from crimescene, but where eyewitness evidence suggests the offender was from a different ethnic group than the suspect, are explored in Champod *et al.* (2004).

11.2 Verbal equivalence of the likelihood ratio

A likelihood ratio is an unambiguous and easily interpretable quantity which expresses the persuasive power of evidence. Nevertheless it can be difficult for those not used to dealing with such quantities to apprehend in some intuitive way the meaning of statements such as 'it is 265 times more likely that the evidence would be observed were the suspect the perpetrator then were some other person the perpetrator'. Even in Western societies where the lay population is used to dealing with notions of probabilities in their day-to-day lives the temptation to transpose the above statement to 'it is 265 more likely that the suspect is the perpetrator than some other person' is overwhelming as the probabilities with which people are used to dealing are probabilities for outcomes, not probabilities for evidence given hypotheses.

Robertson and Vignaux (1995) recommend that a type of scheme in a likelihood ratio is reported as an increase in support for whichever way the evidence points over the impression left by the other evidence in the mind of those whose task it is to decide the ultimate issue. They also recommend, if opportunity presents itself, the use of a sensitivity table, reproduced as Table 11.1, and the reporting of odds rather than probabilities.

Table 11.1 Sensitivity table showing the effect of a likelihood ratio of 1000 on various prior odds. From Robertson and Vignaux (1995) p. 55

prior odds	likelihood ratio	posterior odds
1 to 10	1000	100 to 1
2 to 10	1000	200 to 1
5 to 10	1000	500 to 1
1 to 1	1000	1000 to 1

This scheme has much to commend it as it places a probabilistic argument in the language of the racetrack and betting, a framework in which lay persons are likely to be comfortable. However, reporting an increase in support would absolutely necessitate the use of odds rather than probabilities as otherwise confusion might arise because any reasonable person may start with a probability of 1% of guilt in any trial, and after the evidence is reported which, say, has a likelihood ratio of 265 as above, might lead the same person to conclude that it was almost certain that the defendant was guilty.

Great efforts have been made to express a likelihood ratio on a verbal scale. Table 11.2 is from Evett (1987) based on an outline by Jefferys (1983).

Table 11.2 Verbal scales for likelihood ratios. The equivalents are given in terms of increase in support for C, for likelihood ratios less than 1 take the reciprocal, the equivalent is then support for the complementary hypothesis. The values are on a logarithmic scale. . . . hence go 3.1, 31.6, From Evett (1987)

likelihood ratio	verbal equivalent
$1 < LR \leq 3.1$	slight increase in support for C
$3.1 < LR \leq 31.6$	increase in support for C
$31.6 < LR \leq 316.2$	great increase in support for C
$316.2 < LR$	very great increase in support for C

With the upsurge during the period 1987 to 1998 in reporting likelihood ratios from DNA cases the verbal equivalence scale had to be rewritten to account for some of the very high values encountered. Table 11.3 is a 1998 reformulation of Table 11.2 (Evett, 1998).

However, even the equivalent scale in Table 11.3 was not sufficient to keep up with the range of likelihood ratios encountered in case work, so in 2000 Table 11.3 was revised to Table 11.4 taken from Evett et al. (2000b).

How long constant revisions to a verbal scale for likelihood ratios are to continue is open to debate. It could be that now 'high value' DNA type evidence has been taken into account the scales may have reached a period of stability. However, with the development of more DNA techniques it is possible that there will be an increase

Table 11.3 Verbal scales for likelihood ratios. The equivalents are given in terms of increase in support for C, for likelihood ratios less than 1 take the reciprocal, the equivalent is then support for the complementary hypothesis. From Evett (1998)

likelihood ratio	verbal equivalent
$1 < \text{LR} \leq 10$	limited support for C
$10 < \text{LR} \leq 100$	moderate support for C
$100 < \text{LR} \leq 1000$	strong support for C
$1000 < \text{LR}$	very strong support for C

Table 11.4 Verbal scales for likelihood ratios. The equivalents are given in terms of increase in support for C, for likelihood ratios less than 1 take the reciprocal, the equivalent is then support for the complementary hypothesis. From Evett *et al.* (2000b)

likelihood ratio	verbal equivalent
$1 < \text{LR} \leq 10$	limited support for C
$10 < \text{LR} \leq 100$	moderate support for C
$100 < \text{LR} \leq 1000$	moderately strong support for C
$1000 < \text{LR} \leq 10000$	strong support for C
$10000 < \text{LR}$	very strong support for C

in reported likelihood ratios, hence the continuing need for a verbal scale which will encompass them.

The underlying problem is that although the likelihood ratio of 1 means 'no evidence to support' and always will, there is not a theory of correspondence between number and qualitative description. Also, the qualitative description is itself relativistic and constantly changing dependent on the latest developments in forensic science itself.

A way in which many of the problems encountered with more conventional equivalence schemes is to use some form of equivalence which is in itself comparative. Such a scheme may be to collect many instances of likelihood ratios associated with their respective evidence types and circumstances of collection. When the evidential value of some form of forensic evidence is communicated to lay persons, some other forms of forensic evidence which have similar likelihood ratios can also be presented so that those unfamiliar with using numerical quantities to evaluate evidence can think about the evidence before them in some relative sense. For instance, the appearance of a certain type of glass fragment on a suspect's clothing may have a similar likelihood ratio associated with it to the evidence of a footmark made by a fairly common shoe type in similar circumstances. This may provide a suitable framework by which the observer, unfamiliar with likelihood ratios, can gain some insight into how persuasive the evidence is in the particular case in which they are expected to evaluate that evidence.

There are problems with the scheme outlined above. It can hardly be said to be more consistent than any of the others, and would have difficulty admitting new 'high value' evidence types as there would be no existing comparative material. Most problematic though would be the fact that likelihood ratios are dependent upon the hypotheses under which they are evaluated, and unless the hypotheses from each case in the comparative set of likelihood ratios were similar the comparisons would not be valid.

It is clear that differing individuals will need different ways of explaining a likelihood ratio as a 'strength of evidence'. So the more modes available to those needing to convey the meaning of any statistical evaluation to a lay audience, whether as an increase in support given in odds form, a verbal equivalent of evidential strength, or a comparison to other evidence, the more likely it is that a wider range of people will be able to work with statistical evaluations of forensic evidence.

11.3 Some common criticisms of statistical approaches

The statistical evaluation of evidence explicated and propounded in this volume is termed by some forensic scientists the Bayesian approach, because the core mathematical theory is Bayes' theorem. However, the methods themselves are not necessarily very Bayesian as once it is proposed a likelihood ratio is a suitable measure of the 'value of evidence', Bayes' theorem does not feature too highly in any analysis. Despite this, the approach comes in for criticism, some well-founded, some based on misconceptions, but none with any basis in mathematical theory.

One of the misconceptions which makes its way into the literature is the fact that any 'Bayesian' analysis means that a prior probability has to be established, and by implication the point of the analysis is to establish a posterior probability for guilt of the individual (Kind, 1994; Roberts and Zuckerman, 2004). As we have seen from Sections 9.2 and 9.8 the object of evidence evaluation is to calculate a likelihood ratio which, in Bayes' theorem, changes a prior probability to a posterior probability. We say this is the value of the evidence in the light of those propositions constructed by both the prosecution and defence. This does not necessarily entail that other members of the court should use Bayes' theorem to calculate the probability of guilt or innocence. They may if they wish, but it is not for the statistician or forensic scientist, or anyone else for that matter, to know what processes jurors use to arrive at their conclusions. An evaluation of the evidence is just that, it gives a rationally constructed 'value' by which evidence, usually physical evidence, can be compared with other evidence, and how much evidence 'speaks' of either proposition. If viewed through a Bayesian framework a likelihood ratio has additional very precisely defined meanings in context with all the other evidence in any case, but a likelihood ratio measure of the strength of evidence can just as easily be employed simply without the full paraphernalia of a Bayesian approach.

A consequence of thinking that a prior probability for a defendant's guilt and innocence has to be defined in a completely Bayesian analysis of the evidence is that the defendant cannot be presumed innocent (Kind, 1994). The principle of 'presumption of innocence', has been interpreted to mean that the accused is always innocent until proven guilty. That is, a prior probability of zero should be assigned to the proposition that the accused is guilty. From Equation 22 on p. 109, if we insert 0, and H is the proposition of guilty, then for $\Pr(H)$ it is easy to see that whatever the magnitude of $\Pr(E \mid H)$ and $\Pr(E)$, $\Pr(H \mid E)$ will always stubbornly remain equal to 0. However, the object of evidence evaluation is *not* the establishment of a probability of guilt or innocence, it is the evaluation of the weight of evidence in terms of a pair of propositions put forward by the defence and the prosecution. As has been discussed in Chapter 10, the propositions themselves often do not relate in any direct logical way to the ultimate questions of guilt or innocence, so how a statistical evaluation of evidential strength is expected to do so is difficult to imagine.

A more measured criticism of Bayesian based evidence evaluation methods proposed here is that the databases from which data must be drawn to estimate frequencies for the types of objects which feature in forensic science are simply not available. This would imply that were one to ask an expert examiner on any piece of forensic evidence about the frequency of a particular type of forensic entity in which they had expertise, they would have to reply that they had absolutely no idea whatsoever. The reality is that any expert examiner will have some sort of idea about the frequency of an evidence type about which they have expertise, and should be able to furnish some sort of an answer to the question, even if the answer is vague. This illustrates the fact that there is a database, but the database is informal, and drawn from the expert examiners' experience with the object type in question, rather than a more structured and quantitative survey of the material in question. This sort of estimate of frequency is still an estimate based on a database, even if that database resides in the mental processes of the expert. It would not be ideal, nor desirable, to use such an estimate to evaluate a key piece of evidence in a major criminal trial, however, even these types of frequency estimates can be useful in processes such as sensitivity analysis. Except in a trial such as the Collins case, where the required frequency was for an African male with a beard and moustache, and Caucasian female, the couple possessing a yellow car in Los Angeles (Fairley and Mosteller; 1977 p 355–379), most evidence types will have some sort of accurately estimated frequency. The database criticism is not solely the province of the Bayesian approaches. One does not have to invoke logic beyond the commonsensical to realize that a evidence types for which no estimate of the frequencies involved can be made can have no evaluation attached to them whatsoever beyond speculation.

A better criticism is that, in practice, only single strands of evidence will be evaluated by any single expert examiner. It is unlikely that the expert will be able to examine the rest of the evidence for the case. If another piece of evidence were to be evaluated by numerical means, by some other expert, who did not know about the existence of the first piece of evidence, then were the two pieces of evidence dependent on one another, a court could be severely misled as to the combined value of the two pieces of evidence as they would be presented to the court as though they were independent. At the time of writing it is unlikely that this train of events would happen as case work for forensic statisticians tends to be single strands of more awkward evidence types, the courts beings left to evaluate other evidence in some other way. As more and more evidence types are becoming amenable to evaluation, and demand for the evaluation of forensic evidence is increasing so that, in some criminal trials, several different evidence types may be evaluated by different experts. Again, as with many of the other criticisms levelled at Bayesian approaches this is a problem common to all evidence evaluation, and has to be overcome by members of the court, who will see all the evidence, realizing that two pieces of evidence which are not independent have been treated as though they are, and suitable measures taken to take account of the dependency. Of course the measures taken would involve at some level the introduction of fully conditioned databases for odd combinations of variables (Hodgson, 2002), which, as seen with the Collins case (Fairley and Mosteller, 1977 p 355–379), are unlikely to exist.

If databases and dependency between variables are seen as a barrier to the use of Bayesian approaches and to the evaluation of forensic evidence, it is not because Bayesian methods are uniquely demanding in their data requirements. All conceivable methods of evidence evaluation will place the same demands on forensic scientists to generate data to populate databases; Bayesian methods with their ability to take dependence seriously make this requirement explicit. Any methods for scientific evidence evaluation which promise not to make any demands for data of some sort belong to the realm of speculation, and one would hope criminal and civil courts in any jurisdiction would shy away from them.

Scientific evidence should adhere to the same standards of clarity and public openness of precise measurement that other forms of scientific empirical investigation have always held to be at the core of their methods. Statistical analysis of data which is subject to uncertainty has been a part of that effort since the seventeenth century. If forensic scientists and courts are not to evaluate evidence numerically (Wiersema, 2001) and statistically, where that evidence is amenable to this sort of analysis, then one must ask how this evidence is to be approached? Statistical evaluation, and particularly Bayesian methods such as the calculation of likelihood ratios, have been criticized, but they are the only demonstrably rational means of quantifying the value of evidence available at the moment: anything else is just intuition and guesswork.

12 Evidence evaluation examples

This Section is devoted to some of the simpler practical applications of statistical evaluation of evidence. Most of the examples given here are based upon actual case work which has been undertaken by statisticians working on forensic problems. Although some aspects of each case have been simplified, and the data themselves have been modified to disguise the details of the case involved, the essential thought behind the solutions is the same. The application of evidential evaluation is not always able to conform to strict practice where it is assumed frequencies are known absolutely, and that populations can be sampled without bias. In practice some lateral thinking may be required, and common sense decisions needed about classification of objects to obtain suitable populational frequencies. In some actual cases, but not the ones detailed here, absolutely nothing can be done using statistical analysis to assist the court in its deliberations.

12.1 Blood group frequencies

A domestic burglary had been committed some years ago in New Zealand, and at the time a it was thought the perpetrator had cut themselves on a piece of glass broken during entry to the premises. The blood from the glass was of type O in the ABO system of blood grouping, but the fragment of glass has subsequently been lost, so no DNA can be recovered. Recently the police have arrested a suspect for this offence, that suspect also having blood group of type O. What is the value of the match between the blood found at the scene of the crime and that of the suspect?

Background data

From Buckleton *et al.* (1987) the following frequencies for the components of the ABO system were recorded for New Zealand at around the time of the offence:

Analysis

Although the use of blood group evidence has been replaced to a large degree by DNA in recent years, particularly low copy number DNA, in cases such as this, where items may have been lost, it can still be of value[*].

We have few details about the glass from which the blood was recovered, we also have no statement from the suspect. So it is difficult to formulate any specific proposition about the presence of the blood on the glass, or how the suspect explains, if at all, the bloods presence.

Provisionally we shall assume there is no other explanation for the presence of the blood on the glass other than it got there when the glass was being broken, and that the glass was broken during the burglary, so we assume a link between the blood and the offender.

In the absence of any explanation from the suspect, a provisional defence proposition might be an argument based around complete innocence, that is the suspect was never near the burgled premises, and that the suspect is not the source of the blood.

It would be safer to formulate the prosecution proposition as a source level proposition, simply that H_p is *that the blood is of type O because its source was the suspect*. However, dependent on the actual context in which the blood on the glass was recovered H_p could just as well be given as an activity level proposition. For instance were the glass from the remains of the pane left in the frame, and other information suggested the pane was not broken prior to the burglary.

As we have no other information let H_p be the proposition that: *the source of the blood was the suspect*. As there is no stated defence case a provisional one is at the same level, and is H_d *the source of the blood was someone other than the suspect*.

The value of the evidence, from Equation 27, is:

$$LR = \frac{Pr(E|H_p)}{Pr(E|H_d)}.$$

The numerator is the probability of observing blood group type O on the ABO system given the source of the blood was the suspect. As the suspect has only a single blood type, and that blood type is type O then were the suspect the source of the blood then it is inevitable that the blood recovered from the glass would be of type O, that is $Pr(E|H_p) = 1$.

The denominator in the equation above is the probability of observing the blood to be of type O were the source someone other than the suspect. Were this the case then the probability of observing blood of type O would be the same as observing blood type O from the general population of New Zealand. From Table 12.1 type O occurs with a probability of 0.683. So $Pr(E|H_d) = 0.683$.

---

[*] Barclay *pers. comm.*

Table 12.1 Frequencies of the *ABO* system from New Zealand from Buckleton *et al.* (1987). Reproduced with permission.

Blood group	*A*	*B*	*A B*	*O*
Percentage	25.4%	6.3%	0.0%	68.3%

Therefore:

$$\text{LR} = \frac{1}{0.683}$$
$$= 1.464$$

So the value of this evidence is ≈ 1.5. This may be interpreted as the evidence is 1.5 times as likely if the suspect were the source of the blood, than were someone other than the suspect the source of the blood.

Out of interest, suppose the blood group found on the window was type *B* in the *ABO* system. What is the value of this match?

Proceeding in the same way as with the type *O* blood we find:

$$\text{LR} = \frac{1}{0.063}$$
$$= 15.87$$

Conclusions

The evidence of the observation of blood type *O* in this particular case is ≈ 1.5 as likely were the suspect the source of the blood than someone other than the suspect in the New Zealand population at around the time the offence was committed. The comparison of blood type *O* with type *B* is interesting in that the value of the evidence would be much higher due to the rarity of bloodtype *B* in the *ABO* system. Neither likelihood ratios provide anything other than weak supporting evidence for the prosecution proposition.

This example is the use of value of evidence at its simplest. It assesses a single piece of evidence, with a numerator of 1 and a denominator equivalent to the frequency of the blood group in the population. The value of the evidence goes up with a rarer blood group which is in accords with intuition.

12.2 Trouser fibres

Some fibres had been found on a car seat said to have been involved in a crime committed in New Zealand. The fibres matched a pair of cotton/acrylic trousers in the possession of the suspect. Enquiries revealed the fibres were unique to the type of trousers, and that those trousers had only been made in cuts suitable for men. What is the evidential value of the fibres?

Background data

According to the manufacturers only 12 100 pairs of the specific cotton/acrylic trousers had been imported to New Zealand. A search had been made of the suspect's wardrobe which turned up 3 pairs of denim trousers and a pair of suit trousers in addition to the matching trousers. Survey information suggest that a mean number of trousers for each man is 7, and there are 1.49 million[†] men living in New Zealand.

Analysis

The nature of the criminal activity is unspecified, but presumably the fact that the car is associated in some way with it makes those who have been associated with the car also associated with the offence. The evidence of fibres cannot tell us anything about the offence, and has limited potential to inform us whether the fibres had appeared as a result of sitting contact, slight contact, or secondary transfer. Further information about the numbers and location on the seat may suggest a more specific form of activity, but in the absence of other information it might be wisest to formulate propositions at a source level.

Let H_p be the source level proposition that *the source of the fibres on the car seat is the pair of cotton/acrylic trousers belonging to the suspect*. The corresponding defence proposition again has to be assumed, and, without further information, H_d is that *some pair of trousers other than those belonging to the suspect were the source of the fibres*.

As before the evidence shall be evaluated using a likelihood ratio:

$$LR = \frac{\Pr(E|H_p)}{\Pr(E|H_d)}.$$

First dealing with the numerator. Under H_p the suspect has one pair of trousers from his wardrobe of five pairs which could have left the fibres at the crime scene. We have no reason to suspect that the suspect had any preferences for one pair of trousers in their collection over another, so we shall assume that each pair of trousers is equally likely to be worn. Therefore there is a probability of $1/5 = 0.2$ of seeing fibres from those trousers were the trousers which left the fibres on the car seat those which belonged to the suspect.

The denominator is more difficult. Were the trousers belonging to the suspect not the source of the fibres on the car seat then, assuming that visitors to New Zealand would not have contributed substantially to the population of the particular trouser type, the trousers which left the fibres must have been from one of the other 12 099 pairs of these trousers available in New Zealand. There are 1.49 million men, each with on average 7 pairs of trousers, this makes ≈ 10.4 million pairs of trousers from which the 12 099 were selected. So the probability of seeing fibres from that type of trousers were the defence proposition true is $12,099/10.4 \times 10^6 = 0.001155$.

[†] CIA World Factbook 2002.

Dividing the numerator by the denomonatot gives a likelihood ratio of LR = $0.2/0.001155 \approx 173$, which can be interpreted as the observation of those fibres at the crimescene is ≈ 173 times as likely were the trousers in the possession of the suspect the source of the fibres than were the source of the fibres some pair of trousers not belonging to the suspect.

There must also be some question as to whether trousers are the only potential source of fibres on car seats, and whether men's trousers are the proper population from which the cotton/acrylic trousers are drawn. Fibres on car seats could come from a variety of sources, it could be that the numbers and position of fibres suggests strongly that the fibres came from a lower garment, but could a lower garment equally well be a skirt, or some pair of women's trousers? We have data on men's trousers, and this represents a lower bound for the population from which fibres on seats could be drawn. Hence the likelihood ratio of ≈ 173 is a lower bound of which we can be fairly sure. It is possible that a more realistic likelihood ratio could be calculated based on a population including all lower garments, or indeed, dependent on the arrangement of the fibres on the seat, all garments.

Let us say the fibres found at the crimescene were denim. Further survey information suggests that 60% of trousers in New Zealand are made from denim.

Following the same reasoning as above the numerator is now $3/5 = 0.6$ as the suspect has 5 pairs of trousers, of which 3 are made from denim.

Were the trousers which left the denim fibres not those of the suspect, then the number of trousers that could have left them is $1.49 \times 10^6 \times 7 \approx 10.4$ million total pairs in New Zealand, of which $6/10^{\text{ths}}$ are denim. The 3 pairs contributed by the suspect can be neglected. These are selected from $1.49 \times 10^6 \times 7$ trousers total. So the denominator is:

$$\Pr(E \mid H_d) = \frac{1.49 \times 10^6 \times 7 \times 0.60}{1.49 \times 10^6 \times 7}$$

$$= 0.60$$

So the value of the trouser fibres in the case of denim fibres is:

$$\text{LR} = \frac{0.6}{0.6} = 1.00$$

Which as the LR = 1 means that the evidence is equally likely were the suspect's trousers the source of the car seat fibres or some pair of trousers not belonging to the suspect the source of the fibres. This means the evidence of observing denim in this particular case is of no probative value whatsoever, and incidentally is an illustration of why fibres examiners often disregard denim fibres found at crimescenes.

Conclusions

The likelihood ratio of 173 is moderate supporting evidence that the fibres recovered from the car seat were derived from the pair of cotton/acrylic trousers belonging to the suspect rather than trousers belonging to someone other than the suspect. This assumes that the suspect was equally likely to wear the specific cotton/acrylic trousers as any of the other pairs of trousers available to him, and that the garment leaving the fibres was a pair of men's trousers. This may, dependent on circumstances, be a lower bound about which we can be sure, and the underestimate is of benefit to the defence case. A more realistic likelihood ratio might be calculated by relaxing the assumption that it was a pair of men's trousers which was the source of the fibres recovered from the car seat.

Were the trousers made from denim the picture changes. The resulting likelihood ratio is dependent on the number of denim trousers available to the suspect. Were all of the suspect's trousers denim the the value of the evidence would be $1/0.6 = 1.67$. Were only one of the suspects trousers denim then the value would be $0.2/0.6 = 0.33$, which would weakly suggest the suspects innocence. Either way fibres which could only be associated with denim trousers would be of little probative value in this case.

12.3 Shoe types

A burglary has been committed in Bradford-upon-Avon. On a window sill a footmark was found, which when developed was unmistakably made by a Wellborn Stripe training shoe. There is no evidence that anyone other than the intruder had cause to stand on the window sill. A suspect was identified and detained. The suspect's residence was searched and six pairs of shoes were found which included two pairs of Wellborn Stripe training shoes and a pair of football boots. Cut marks found on one of the pairs of Wellborn trainers were seen to clearly match that of the crimescene mark, there being no differences between the print made by the suspect's shoe and the mark developed from the crimescene. What is the evidential value of the footmark?

Background data

A representative from Wellborn says that 35 000 pairs of the Stripe trainer were sold in the United Kingdom. Table 12.2 was obtained from enquiries with the British Footwear Association and the Office of National Statistics (United Kingdom).

Analysis

With the information that the crimescene footmark was found on the window ledge of a property, and no innocent explanation of how such a mark might get to the particular place, an activity level of proposition, rather than a source level, may be appropriate. However, from the point of view of the expert witness source level propositions may be epistomologically safer. Allowing the court to make the inference to the activity level. A suitable prosecution proposition H_p could be: *the shoe which made the shoemark at the crimescene belongs to the suspect.* A defence proposition is again

Table 12.2 Footwear sales in the United Kingdom during 2003 by type of footwear. Sales are in millions of pairs. This is a subsection of the full dataset provided by British Footwear Association and the Office of National Statistics (United Kingdom). Types considered suitable for the purpose of entering a house by the author are marked*.

Type (description)	Sales
Waterproof footwear with rubber uppers non-safety	2.5
Waterproof footwear with plastic uppers non-safety	3.7
Sandals with rubber or plastic outer soles and uppers	16
Town footwear with rubber or plastic uppers	37*
Slippers and other indoor footwear with plastic uppers	1.3
Men's town footwear with leather uppers including boots	30.2*
Women's town footwear with leather uppers including boots	55.7
Children's town footwear with leather uppers including boots	20.8
Footwear with rubber, plastic or leather outer soles and textile uppers excluding slippers, other indoor footwear and sports footwear	30*

absent, and will have to be provisional and assumed. The corresponding defence proposition H_d could be: *the shoe which made the shoemark at the crimescene was not made by one of the shoes belonging to the suspect*. Notice the above propositions do not imply that the suspect was wearing the shoes at the time of the offence, that is a fact for the court to decide, the evidence can only tell us anything about shoes. The propositions stated here also carefully avoid suggesting anything about the number of individuals involved in entering the domicile, and that the evidence as it is cannot tell us whether the individual who entered the premises actually committed the offence of burglary. It has to be left for the court to decide whether the individual who entered the house was a person involved in the burglary.

As before the value of this evidence, from Equation 27, is expressed as the likelihood ratio:

$$LR = \frac{Pr(E|H_p)}{Pr(E|H_d)}.$$

First let us consider the numerator. We are told that the suspect had six pairs of shoes in total, two of which were Wellborn Stripe shoes, the same shoe type which left the mark at the crimescene. The numerator asks *what is the probability of observing a Wellborn Stripe footwear mark given that a pair of the suspect's shoes made the mark?* There is no evidence to suggest the suspect favours wearing one particular pair of their shoes, so we shall assume that there is an equal probability that each pair of the suspect's shoes would have been worn. As the suspect has six pairs of shoes, two of which are indistinguishable from the mark found at the crimescene $Pr(E|H_p) = 2/6 = 1/3$.

The denominator is the probability of observing a Wellborn Stripe shoe given that the crimescene mark was made by a shoe other than the Wellborn Stripe shoe belonging to the suspect. First we must define a suitable population of potential suspect shoes. As this is a burglary, and without any information to the contrary, the most appropriate population might be that of pairs of shoes in Bradford on Avon. However Table 12.2 gives us data for the United Kingdom as a whole, not for Bradford on Avon, and the 35 000 pairs of Welborn Stripe shoes is for the United Kingdom. So we cannot directly know the frequency of observing a Wellborn Stripe shoe in Bradford on Avon, but we can calculate it for the United Kingdom. If it is thought that the frequency of Wellborn Stripe shoes amongst the population of shoes is any different to that of the United Kingdom then data for sales in Bradford on Avon must be obtained. If on the other hand it is reasonable to suggest that the proportion of Wellborn Stripe shoes in Bradford on Avon is no different to that of the rest of the United Kingdom then the data for the United Kingdom may be used as a basis from which to calculate the frequency of Wellborn Stripe shoes in Bradford on Avon. In the absence of other information we shall assume there is no reason to think that Bradford on Avon is any different to the United Kingdom in respect of its distribution of shoe types.

The next problem is from which population of shoe types are the Wellborn Stripe shoes detected at the crimescene selected. For instance, is it reasonable when selecting a population of shoes to include footwear which could not possibly be used, such as football boots, and spiked running shoes. The probability of observing the Wellborn Stripe shoes is that of observing them drawn from a population of shoes in which it would be at least possible to perform the activity of entering the premises. This brings in the notion of "fit for purpose". Such footwear as skiing boots might not be considered fit for the purpose of entering a house via a window, therefore might not be considered as being amongst the possible footwear. From Table 12.2 the categories which are waterproof plastic or rubber footwear sound as though they include Wellington boots, thus might not be suitable. The same is true of all categories of children's footwear and sandals. The categories of town shoes with leather, plastic or textile uppers would be considered suitable. However womens shoes might include raised platform shoes and those with stiletto heels which would certainly not be suitable for the purpose of entering. In Table 12.2 those types considered suitable are marked with an *. There were 97.2 million of these sold in the United Kingdom in 2003.

Should there not be more shoes in the whole of the United Kingdom from which the Wellborn Stripe shoes detected from the crimescene mark could have been detected? Actually yes, the actual population would be many more. The sales figures in Table 12.2 are restricted to 2003. It is reasonable to say that most of the shoes which were sold in 2003 would be part of the United Kingdom population of shoes at the end of 2003. But there would also be shoes in the population from previous years. Just how many it is not possible from the data we have, so it is likely that the 97.2 million pairs of shoes estimates above is a gross underestimate of the true numbers of pairs of footwear in which it would be possible to enter a house via the window. It is, however, an underestimate at which we can be reasonably sure, and being an underestimate favours the defence case.

We know there are 35 000 pairs of Wellborn Stripe shoes in the United Kingdom, 34 998 not belonging to the suspect, and a minimum of 97.2 million pairs of shoes from which any of those pairs could have been selected. So there is a probability of $34\,998/97.3 \times 10^6 = 0.00036$ of observing a shoemark and it being that made by a Wellborn Stripe shoe. This forms the denominator.

The likelihood ratio for this evidence is therefore:

$$LR = \frac{1/3}{0.00036}$$
$$= 925.92$$

We have been told that one of the suspect's pairs of shoes had acquired features which made it indistinguishable from that mark recovered from the burgled house. Is there anything we can do with this further information? We have been told that there are 35 000 pairs of Wellborn Stripe shoes sold in the United Kingdom. How far do the acquired features go to narrowing the population of these particular shoes? Without further data on the acquisition of features during use it is not possible to say. Some types of shoe will be particularly vulnerable to developing wear and split features on the soles due to design and manufacturing details, others features may be a consequence of random factors. Without a study of these features and the frequencies with which they occur amongst the specific type of shoe it is not possible to offer any further quantification for this evidence. However, what can be said is that as the acquired features are not seen on every Wellborn Stripe training shoe the number of Wellborn Stripe shoes exactly matching that of the mark found at the crimescene may be considerably lower than the 35 000 pairs of shoes in the Wellborn Stripe population. Hence the likelihood ratio taking the acquired features into account might be very much higher than that calculated above. How much greater is impossible to calculate without further data.

Conclusions

The calculated likelihood ratio of ≈ 926 represents the value of the evidence. It has been assumed that:

- the prosecution proposition is that the footmark found at the crimescene was made by one of the shoes belonging to the suspect.

- The defence proposition is: the shoe which made the shoemark found at the crimescene was made by a shoe belonging to someone other than the suspect.

- The suspect uses each pair of their shoes equally.

- The proportion of Wellborn Stripe shoes in Bradford on Avon is no different to that of the United Kingdom.

The likelihood ratio given above is an underestimate of the true value of this evidence. The underestimate being due to the fact that the population from which the particular shoe type was selected was estimated using data from only 2003, and the 35 000 pairs of Welborn Stripe shoes were the total number of those particular shoes sold. It is almost certain that the actual population of shoes would be larger because many shoes from previous years should be included in the population estimate, though how many this would be is impossible to calculate using the data here. Additionally, it has not been possible to calculate the effect of the acquired features seen on both crimescene mark and suspects shoe. To examine the effects of acquired features would require additional data and expert knowledge of the wear characteristics of this type of shoe.

12.4 Airweapon projectiles

A projectile has been recovered from an incident involving an airweapon attack on the property of an elderly person. The examiners in the firearms section say that the projectile is a lead pellet, and from a rifled barrel with wide lands and narrow grooves. The calibre of the pellet is 0.25, which the firearms examiners consider unusual. Deformation and barrel wear mean that there are no further distinguishing marks upon the pellet. There are no differences between it and one recovered from a similar incident a few months before in an adjoining housing estate. What is the value of the evidence that the two projectiles were fired from the same weapon?

Background data

Table 12.3 features some (simulated) firearm data taken from the previous five years.

Table 12.3   Data from firearm incidents (simulated) from the previous five years.

number of shootings	22
number of incidents involving airweapons	38
Athena airweapons seized	8
Walker airifles seized	5
unidentified firearms seized	12
shotguns seized	8
AJS airweapons seized	11
Thor airweapons seized	2
Williamson airweapons seized	3
boxes of pellets seized	56

Firearms examiners after referring to Smith (1978) say that the narrow rifling grooves and wide lands indicate the weapon used was a Walker airweapon. Enquiries with Walkers reveal that of 2 154 000 airweapons made by them only 11 880 were of 0.25 calibre, the calibre now being considered obsolete.

Analysis

In this case the respective propositions are relatively simple to formulate as the question is one which is asked solely as a matter of intelligence, and not involving some possibly complex alternative explanation for the evidence. H_p is *the pellets recovered from the two incidents were fired from the same weapon*, H_d being *the pellets recovered from the two incidents were fired from different weapons*.

The evidential value will be expressed as the likelihood ratio:

$$LR = \frac{Pr(E|H_p)}{Pr(E|H_d)}.$$

The numerator is the probability of observing the evidence give that the pellets from the two incidents were fired from the same weapon. The evidence E has two components A, the pellet has narrow grooves and wide lands, and, B, the pellet is of 0.25 calibre. The numerator can therefore be rewritten $Pr(A, B|H_p)$. Were the two pellets fired from the same weapon then one would expect that these two pieces of information should match if the weapon has not been re-barrelled in the intervening period. Assume that, were a single weapon used in both incidents, it would be extremely unlikely that the barrel would have been modified. So $Pr(A, B|H_p) = 1$.

The denominator can be rewritten $Pr(A, B|H_d)$ which is the probability of the pellet having wide lands and narrow grooves **and** of 0.25 calibre were different weapons used in the separate incidents. Which using the third law of probability (discussed on page 20) can be stated:

$$Pr(A, B|H_d) = Pr(A|H_d) \times Pr(B|A, H_d)$$

where $Pr(A|H_d)$ is the probability of observing narrow grooves and wide lands were the weapons used in the two incidents not the same weapon, and is equivalent to observing a weapon with narrow grooves and wide lands from the population of weapons. And $Pr(B|A, H_d)$ is the probability of observing a calibre of 0.25 **given** that we have observed a weapon with narrow grooves and wide lands. The observation "narrow grooves and wide lands" our experts tell us is equivalent to saying that the weapon was made by Walker.

The next problem is what is the appropriate population of weapons from which the weapon(s) used in the two incidents was/were selected? It might be considered appropriate to think that the weapon(s) were selected from all projectile weapons were the attacks on people, but the circumstances of the incidents would indicate a more nuisance type of attack upon property the perpetrators of which would probably not have access to conventional firearms. So provisionally the population from which the weapon(s) was/were selected will be all airweapons.

From the information suppled there have been 29 air weapons seized in the last five years, 5 of which were made by Walker. If the unseen population of airweapons is no different to the seized population of airweapons then the probability of observing an airweapon and it being made by Walker is 5/29 = 0.17. So $\Pr(A|H_d) = 0.17$.

$\Pr(B|A, H_d)$ is the probability of observing an airweapon of 0.25 calibre **given** it has been made by Walker. Walker said that of 2 154 000 airweapons made by them only 11 880 were of 0.25 calibre, so $\Pr(B|A, H_d) = 11880/2154000 = 0.0055$.

Multiplying the two parts of the denominator $0.17 \times 0.0055 = 0.0009$. So the likelihood ratio is $1/0.0009 \approx 1070$.

Conclusions

By assuming that the proportion of Walker airweapons amongst seized airweapons is the same as that in the wider population of airweapons, and that were the same weapon used in the two incidents the barrel was not modified, a likelihood ratio of 1070 has been calculated. This is for the evidence of observing that the rifling pattern is of narrow grooves and wide lands, and that the calibre of the pellet was 0.25, for the propositions: H_p, the pellets were fired from the same weapon; H_d, the pellets fired in the two incidents were fired from different weapons. The evidence provides moderate to strong support for the proposition that the pellets found at the two incidents were fired from the same weapon.

12.5 Height description from an eyewitness

The cashier at a post-office which had recently fallen prey to an armed robbery said she is sure the offender was an adult male, and around 6′ tall. Police have detained a suspect who is 6′1″ tall, and have no reason to suspect the cashier was mistaken in her description of the offender. What is the evidential value of the cashier's description?

Background data

From standard growth tables (Patel *et al.*: 2003) the stature of men in the United Kingdom is 177.5 cm with a standard deviation of 9.76 cm. Further questioning of the eyewitness reveals that "around" 6′ means the eyewitness is 90% sure he was between 5′8″ and 6′3″. The suspect detained by Police is 6′1″ tall.

Analysis

As the eyewitness was a direct witness to the offence, propositions in this case could possibly be at the offence level. However, it is safer to reduce the level to an activity level, or source level. Let H_p be the proposition *the individual described by the cashier was the suspect*, and H_d be *the individual described by the cashier was someone other than the suspect*.

We shall evaluate the stature evidence using the likelihood ratio:

$$LR = \frac{Pr(E|H_p)}{Pr(E|H_d)} \tag{12.1}$$

where $Pr(E|H_p)$ is the probability of observing the suspect's true height given that the suspect is the individual described by the eyewitness, and $Pr(E|H_d)$ is the probability of observing the suspect's true height given the cashier's description was some other man from the United Kingdom population.

The cashier is 90% certain that the individual she saw was between 5′8″ and 6′3″. For simplicity let us work in centimetres. So 5′8″ = 172.7 cm, and 6′3″ = 190.5 cm. The suspect's height is 6′1″ = 185.5 cm.

If we model the eyewitnesses' height description as a normal distribution then the mean is 172.7 + {(190.5 − 172.7)/2} = 181.6. The standard deviation is a little more difficult to work out, but from Appendix B we know that {(190.5 − 172.7)/2} = 8.9 is between 1.64 and 1.65, call it 1.645, standard deviations.[‡] As 8.9 is 1.645 standard deviations then the standard deviation for the eyewitnesses height description is 8.9/1.645 = 5.41 cm.

From here there are two ways of evaluating the likelihood ratio given in Equation 12.1. The first uses what we learned in Section 4 and the tabulated values in Appendix B to evaluate the numerator and denomonator for Equation 12.1, and is an approximate value for the likelihood ratio. The second uses the equation for the normal probability density function, and can be regarded as an exact solution given the assumptions.

1. For the approximate solution refer to Figure 12.1. Figure 12.1 has depicts two normal models, one which describes the observation of the eyewitness (solid line) which has a mean of 181.6 cm and a sd of 5.41 cm. The other normal is that for the male population of the United Kingdom as a whole (dashed line) which has a mean of 177.5 cm and sd of 9.76 cm. The suspects' true height of 185.5 cm.

   The probability of observing the suspects height of 185.5 cm given the eyewitnesses description is indicated on Figure 12.1 and is proportional to the height A. This can be calculated directly, or approximated by the shaded areas area $\alpha + \beta$. For a less accurate approximation it can even be measured directly from the y axis of Figure 12.1.

   The chosen range between which to calculate the area is between 184 cm and 187 cm. This range is arbitrary, and could just as well be smaller or larger, but should be small in relation to the total range of heights.

[‡] Look up 0.95% of the area in the main body of the text. We look up 0.95% because the tabulation in Appendix B is for a single tail on the right, we need to have our 90% area with 5% in each tail.

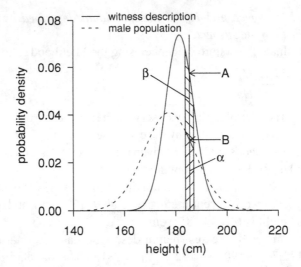

Figure 12.1 The witness uncertainty assuming a normal distribution of mean of 181.6 cm and standard deviation as 5.41 cm given the witness is 90% sure is represented as the solid line. The dotted line superimposed is the normal distribution of heights for adult males. This has mean of 177.5 cm and standard deviation of 9.76 cm. The suspect's height is the solid vertical line at 185.5 cm. The likelihood ratio is given by the ratio of the heights A to B as indicated. These can be read directly from the Figure, or approximated from the shaded areas α and $\alpha + \beta$.

$\alpha + \beta$ is the area under a normal curve with parameters 181.6 cm $\pm$ 5.41 cm between 184 cm and 187 cm, and proportional to the probability of observing the suspects' height were the suspect the individual the cashier saw. 184 cm is at $(184 - 181.6)/5.41 = 0.44$ standard deviations. 187 cm is at $(187 - 181.6)/5.41 = 0.99$ standard deviations. From Appendix B the area under the normal curve up to 0.99 standard deviations is 0.8389, the area under the curve up to 0.44 standard deviations is 0.6700. $0.8389 - 0.06700 = 0.1689$.

The area α in Figure 12.1 is the area under the normal curve with parameters 177.5 cm $\pm$ 9.76 cm between 184 cm and 187 cm, and is proportional to the height B and the probability of observing an individual who is not the suspect, but who has a height of 185.5 cm. 184 cm is at $(184 - 177.5)/9.76 = 0.66$ standard deviations. 187 cm is at $(187 - 177.5)/9.76 = 0.97$ standard deviations. From Appendix B the area under the normal curve up to 0.97 standard deviations is 0.8340, the area under the curve up to 0.66 standard deviations is 0.7454. $0.8340 - 0.7454 = 0.0886$.

Using areas as to find an approximate likelihood ratio we can calculate it as the ratio of the two areas, which is $0.1689/0.0886 = 1.9$.

2. A more exact answer would be to calculate densities A and B directly. The ratio of A to B would then be in the same ratio as the numerator and denominator in Equation 12.1.

To do this we need to know the equation for the normal probability density curve. This is:

$$f(x|\theta, \delta) = \frac{1}{\sqrt{2\pi\delta^2}} \exp\left\{-\frac{(x-\theta)^2}{2\delta^2}\right\} \tag{12.2}$$

where x is the point at which we are trying to calculate the density, θ and δ are the mean and standard deviation of the particular normal distribution that the density corresponding to point x is being calculated. The notation $\exp\{\ldots\}$ may be unfamilier, but simply means $e^{\{\ldots\}}$, where e is 2.718.

The distribution describing the eyewitnesses uncertainty has a mean of 181.6 cm, and standard deviation of 5.41 cm. So we can substitute $\theta = 181.6$, and $\delta = 5.41$ into Equation 12.2. The suspect has a height of 185.5 cm, so we can set $x = 185.5$.

$$f(185.5|\theta = 181.6, \delta = 5.41) = \frac{1}{\sqrt{2\pi(5.41)^2}} \exp\left\{-\frac{(185.5 - 181.6)^2}{2 \times 5.41^2}\right\}$$

$$= \frac{1}{\sqrt{2\pi \times 29.27}} \exp\left\{-\frac{(3.9)^2}{2 \times 29.27}\right\}$$

$$= \frac{1}{\sqrt{183.82}} \exp\left\{-\frac{15.21}{58.54}\right\}$$

$$= \frac{1}{13.56} \exp\{-0.26\}$$

$$= 0.057.$$

An exact value for the numerator in Equation 12.1 can be said to be 0.057.

The denomonator can be calculated in the same way, but using the parameters of the normal distribution describing the heights of the population of men in the United Kingdom. The mean of heights for men was 177.5 cm, the standard deviation was 9.76 cm. Substituting these values into Equation 12.1:

$$f(185.5|\theta = 177.5, \delta = 9.76) = \frac{1}{\sqrt{2\pi(9.76)^2}} \exp\left\{-\frac{(185.5 - 177.5)^2}{2 \times 9.76^2}\right\}$$

$$= \frac{1}{\sqrt{2\pi \times 95.26}} \exp\left\{-\frac{(8)^2}{2 \times 95.26}\right\}$$

$$= \frac{1}{\sqrt{598.54}} \exp\left\{-\frac{64}{190.52}\right\}$$

$$= \frac{1}{24.47} \exp\{-0.336\}$$

$$= 0.029.$$

The numerator is 0.057, and the denomonator is 0.029, so the likelihood ratio is 0.057/0.029 = 1.97

Conclusions

Assuming that the witness' description represents a statement of confidence which can be adequately modelled with a normal distribution of mean 181.6 cm and standard deviation 5.41 cm, a likelihood ratio of 1.97 can be calculated. This can be interpreted as the eyewitnesses description is 1.97 times as likely were the suspect the person being described by the cashier as any other man in the population. This offers slight support for the prosecution proposition that the suspect was the man described by the cashier.

The approximation for the likelihood ratio, calculated from the areas α and β from Figure 12.1, and tabulated values of those areas is 1.9, which is a good approximation for the purposes of evidence evaluation to the more precise calculation of 1.97. However, the more precise calculation would be prefered were this evidence being evaluated in a real case.

13 Errors in interpretation

There are a number of mistakes in interpretation which can lead to evidence being regarded in a misleading light. Broadly errors of interpretator can be divided into those which are based upon a misunderstanding of statistics, and those which are made at a fundamental level of interpretation.

13.1 Statistically based errors of interpretation

These errors of interpretation are based upon some fundamental misunderstanding of probability.

Transposed conditional

This is a very common error in interpretation, and one which can be all too easy to make. In essence the terms $\Pr(E \mid H)$ and $\Pr(H \mid E)$ from Equation 22 on p. 109, that is, the probability of the evidence given the hypothesis, and the probability of the hypothesis given the evidence, are interchanged.

From the example of sex and the presence of the rhomboid fossa in Tables 9.1 and 9.2 on p. 109 the probability that a skeleton from the sample comes from a male given the presence of a rhomboid fossa is 93%, whereas the probability of a skeleton from the sample has a rhomboid fossa given that the skeleton is male is 67%. These are obviously not the same, and really should not be confused.

The fallacy of the transposed conditional, sometimes called the *prosecutor's fallacy* comes in many incarnations. In the bloodgroup example in Section 12.1 on p. 139 the probability of observing the bloodgroup O given the suspect is not the perpetrator, but has bloodgroup O is 0.683, this is not to be read as a 68.3% probability of innocence, hence a 31.7% probability of guilt.

Evett and Weir (1998, p. 30) give a verbal example of this mistake where the courts often require the DNA expert witness to give some measure of the evidential value based on the occurrence of the particular profile in the population at large. The statement *the probability of observing this type of profile from a person other than the suspect is* 1/100 is correct. It makes a statement about the evidence: *this type of profile*, given the hypothesis, *a person other than the suspect*. Evett and Weir (1998, p. 30) relate that a common error would be to transpose the above statement to the probability that this profile came from someone else is 1/100. This is incorrect as it has transposed the statement above to the probability of a proposition, *this profile came from someone else is* 1/100, conditional on a match between the crimescene profile and the suspect's profile.

Evett (1995) suggests: *Do not offer a probability for the truth of a hypothesis* to forensic scientists engaged in report writing. However, it is relatively easy for writers to avoid transposing conditionals if they think about what they are writing. A more difficult task, due to the ambiguities in natural languages, is to understand the conditioning implicit in written reports when reading them.

In their extensive work on human hair Gaudette and Keeping (1974) made multiple comparisons between many different follicles from many different people. In an experiment nine hairs from one person were compared with a hair from a different person. From the results of many such comparison experiments they estimated that the probability that in nine such comparisons at least two hairs would be indistinguishable would be 1/4500. The authors stated:

'it is estimated that if one human scalp hair found at the scene of a crime is indistinguishable from at least one of a group of about nine dissimilar hairs from a given source the probability that it could have originated from another source is very small, about 1/4500'.

Here Gaudette and Keeping's (1974) experiment provides a value for the probability of finding indistinguishable hairs given that the sources are known to be the same, however, their statement above transposes this to the probability of the source of the hairs being different from the comparative material given indistinguishably, which is a common slip in interpretation.

Evett (1995) gives the sound advice, 'If a statement is to be made of probability or odds then it is good practice to use 'if' or 'given' explicitly to clarify the conditioning information', and this would certainly have resolved some of the ambiguity in the statements above.

Defender's fallacy

The fallacy of the transposed conditional has been termed the *prosecutor's fallacy*; a counterpart is the defender's fallacy. Suppose evidence, such as a DNA profile, occurs with a probability of 1%, and the total population from which the offender could be drawn was 10 000. The defence could argue that the evidence would occur in 100 individuals in the population, thus was of little value. There are two problems with this interpretation, first, because the number of suspects has been narrowed from 10 000 to 100, 9900 people have been excluded. This could hardly be the effect of valueless evidence. Secondly, as argued by Evett and Weir (1998, p. 32), it is unlikely that all 100 are equally likely to be guilty.

Another match error

This error mistakes rarity of evidence occurring, and the numbers of occurrences of that evidence in a population. As above, take a genetic marker which occurs with a frequency of 1% in a population of 10 000. The probability of a person selected at random from the population not matching the marker is $1 - 0.01 = 0.99$. If the marker occurs independently in the population, that is, that an occurrence of it in one person makes it no more, or less, likely that it occurs in another, then the probability of the marker occurring in no other individuals is $0.99_1 \times 0.99_2 \times 0.99_i \ldots \times 0.99_{i=10,000} = 0.99^{10,000}$. The complementery probability that there is one, or more, other occurrences of the marker is therefore $1 - 0.99^{10,000} \approx 1$. This means that it is almost certain that a marker occurring with a frequency of 1% will be found in a population of 10 000.

Now let the marker occur with a frequency of 1 in a million, or 0.000001, the probability that the marker does *not* occur in any individual is $1 - 0.000001 = 0.999999$, so the probability that there is no other occurrence in the population of 10 000 is $0.999999^{10,000} \approx 0.99$. Therefore the probability that there is at least a single occurrence of the marker occurring in the population of $10,000$ is $\approx 1\%$.

As the marker occurs with probabilly 0.000001, and the population is only 10 000, the expected frequency of the marker's occurrence is $0.000001 \times 10,000 = 0.01$.

This example illustrates the fact that despite the frequency of the occurrence of some evidence being such that the expected frequency is less than the reciprocal of the population, there is still a non-negligible probability that there is at least one occurrence of the marker in the population.

Numerical conversion error

The numerical conversion errors is a sort of converse to the problem and is 'another match error', seen in statements such as: were a marker were to occur with a frequency of 1% then 100 people would have to be examined to observe the marker. This is an incorrect statement, as were a marker to occur with frequency 0.01 then there would be a certain probability of observing that marker were 100 to be observed. Following the working above, the probability of not observing the marker in any person is $1 - 0.01 = 0.99$, so with independence of the marker, the probability of not observing the marker in 100 observations is 0.99^{100}. Hence the probability of observing the marker from 100 observations is $1 - (0.99^{100}) = 0.63$, or, 63%.

In notation:

$$\Pr(E \mid n) = 1 - (1 - \gamma)^n$$

where γ is the frequency of occurrence, n is the number of observations and E denotes the event of 1 or more occurrences. So to find the minimum number of observations which will result in an observation of the marker with probability of at least P then the following inequality must be satisfied:

$$P \leq 1 - (1 - \gamma)^n$$

$$1 - P \leq (1 - \gamma)^n$$

$$\log(1 - P) \leq n \log 1 - \gamma$$

$$n \geq \frac{\log(1 - P)}{\log(1 - \gamma)} \tag{32}$$

Therefore, were a marker to occur with a frequency of 1×10^{-6} in a population, and we wished to observe it with a probability of 99%, then substituting 0.99 for P, and 1×10^{-6} for γ into Equation 32 we would have to make at least 4.6 million observations.

13.2 Methodological errors of interpretation

These errors of interpretation are errors in the methodology and assumptions applied to any analysis of evidence, and are not contained to statistical evaluations of evidence.

Different level error

The different level error has been mentioned before in Section 8.4. This is where propositions inferred at one level are transferred to another level. For instance, a crime is committed and glass from a particular type of bottle is found at the scene which is of similar chemical composition to that found in the possession of a suspect. This does not test the hypothesis that the two fragments are from the same bottle, merely that the two fragments have chemical compositions which could have come from the same distribution. The value of evidence is mostly related to the rarity of the bottle type.

Broadly speaking, just comparing two objects gives some idea as to whether they are of the same type, or if they are not of the same type. Knowing that two objects are not of the same type can in itself be very valuable information as it allows exclusion, but if a *match* is found it leads to the very weak proposition of some trace evidence 'not excluding' a suspect. Evidence can only be evaluated in any satisfactory manner if a *database* for the population of objects is known. Sometimes an object is very rare, in which case the background frequency of similar objects is very low, and the value of a *match* is high. For more common objects the value of a *match* is lower. However, the value of evidence is decided not only on the similarity between an object found in the possession of a suspect and one found at the scene of a crime, but how many other objects of a similar type exist.

As a thought experiment to illustrate the point above, suppose that ten bottles, of between one and ten different and distinct colours, are broken. A number of fragments are selected from the fragments of each bottle and placed into a bag, one bag for the fragments from each bottle. Imagine a fragment falls onto the floor from one of the ten bags, but we do not know which of the bags it came from. The fragment is red. Suppose it is suspected that the fragment came from a particular bag, so a fragment is drawn from that bag, and it, too, is red. What value has the observation that both fragments are red upon our belief that the two fragments are from the same bottle?

If all ten bottles were of red glass, then the observation that the two fragments were both red would have no value as the probability of drawing a red fragment is 1 regardless of which bag we choose. However, were only one bottle from the ten bottles made of red glass, then the evidential value for the observation 'red glass' would be conclusive that the two fragments were from the same bottle.

From the above it is obvious that the evidential value lies not only in similarity of observation, but also in the relative frequency of the objects being 'matched'. Similarity of properties alone gives no information as to whether trace evidence comes from the same source, but have to be used in conjunction with knowledge of the same properties in the wider population.

Defendant's database fallacy

We have already mentioned the defendant's database fallacy in Section 11.1.2. It revolve around the question of the appropriate database to use when estimation the frequency of any particular observation. For example, suppose a crime has been committed and a fragment of a particular shirt type found in association with the crimescene. If a suspect who is from East London is apprehended and found to have a similar shirt, and no other information about the offender is available, the value of the evidence is related to the frequency of the shirt type amongst top garments in a wider geographical region than East London. If, however, it were known from independent sources that the offender was an East Londoner, then the value of the evidence would be related to the frequency of the shirt type amongst outer garments of people from East London.

Independence assumption

A common error is to assume independence where none exists. A recent and high profile case in a United Kingdom jurisdiction is that of Sally Clark in 1999. A consultant paediatrician gave a probability for observing two sudden infant death syndrome (SIDS) deaths in a single family as 1 in 73 million. The probability of observing a single SIDS death in a family from a similar environment to the Clark's was quoted by him from a study as 1 in 8500. The consultant then treated the two cases as independent, and used the product of two events of the same probability to obtain the 1 in 73 million figure (Watkins, 2001). However, it is not at all clear, without further justification, that the events are independent. SIDS is an as yet unexplained cause of infant mortality. A possible cause is some inherited genetic anomaly. If the the anomaly is inherited then if one child from a set of parents has the anomaly there may be increased chance any other child in the family has it as well were this the case then it would be clearly incorrect to treat there two events as though they were independent. Independence of SIDS deaths within a family is a matter of the science of pediatrics, and requires pheditricians to justify it.

Review questions

1. Why are the conclusions of the following arguments erroneous:

   (a) There is a 1% chance of observing the DNA profile were the defendent innocent, therefore there is a 99% probability the defendent is guilty.
   (b) From binomial theorem there is a 99% probability that there are over 10 000 individuals in the United Kingdom with this blood type. Therefore the evidence is useless as there is only a 1/10 000 probability the suspect is guilty.
   (c) The evidence of a DNA match is 10 000 times as likely were the DNA profile to have come from the suspect as some other individual in the population. Therefore the blood is 10 000 times more likely to have come from the suspect than from someone else.

2. A fleck of paint from a car suspected of being involved in a collision has been found on the other vehicle involved with the collision. The two on the basis of colour and composition match at $\geq 99\%$ confidence; therefore there is $\leq 1\%$ chance that this car was not involved in the collision. How many errors are involved in this interpretation?

3. From Table 3.3 50% of marijuana seizures from 1986 have a Δ^9-THC content between 7% and 8.5%. If the THC content of a seizure from an unknown year is 7.5% would it be true to say that there is a 50% probability it came from 1986? Why?

14 DNA I

The use of DNA as evidence is a relatively recent development in forensic science. First introduced to forensic science in the mid 1980s its discriminating ability is large compared with other evidence types, and has great exculpatory power (Johnson and Williams, 2004) as well as a high level of probative value for the prosecution. The explicitly statistical nature of the interpretation of DNA evidence has led to a demand by courts in various jurisdictions for probabilistic analysis to be applied to other types of forensic evidence. Hence, in some ways the application of DNA techniques has led indirectly to the further development of many of the statistical evidence evaluation methods explored earlier in this book.

14.1 Loci and alleles

A popular form, although by no means the only form, of DNA in forensic science is the short tandem repeat (STR). An STR DNA profile consists of a series of *loci* each with two numbers, or letters, indicating the number of repeated units for each of the alleles present on that loci in the individual who donated the DNA. In inheritance one allele will come from the mother, the other from the father of the individual. For forensic purposes it is usual to report on several loci. The loci are selected by forensic scientists so that they are not functional, that is, these sequences of DNA do not code for any metabolic protein, and so that they are some distance away from each other in the genome.

Çakir *et al.* (2001) collected DNA samples from 80 unrelated individuals from those convicted of offences in Turkey. In their work they examined the TPOX locus and reported on alleles 6, 8, 9, 10, 11, 12. They reported that 25 people had TPOX (8, 11). This means that for the TPOX locus the people who were TPOX (8, 11) could have inherited an allele of eight repeats of the TPOX sequence from their mother or father, and an allele of 11 repeats of the TPOX sequence from their mother or father.

Introduction to Statistics for Forensic Scientists   David Lucy
© 2005 John Wiley & Sons, Ltd.

By observation of the individuals alone it is not possible to tell which allele came from which parent. Even were the TPOX sequences known for the parents it would not always be the case that the exact line of inheritance could be reconstructed.

A TPOX genome of 8 TPOX sequences long and 11 TPOX sequences long, would be referred to as *heterozygous* for TPOX. Çakir *et al.* (2001) also report on 18 individuals who had the TPOX sequence (8, 8), which means both TPOX alleles are 8 repeats long. This is referred to as *homozygosity*.

Above, the sequences for the TPOX loci are known as *genotypes*. A genotype comprises information for both alleles for the locus.

14.2 Simple case genotypic frequencies

In Section 9.3 we discussed how numerical evidence can be given the form of a *value of evidence*. DNA being numerical evidence can also be treated in exactly the same way.

Suppose blood had been recovered from broken glass at a crimescene in Turkey. The genotypes LDLR(A, A), GYPA(A, B), HBGG(B, B), D7S8(A, B) and Gc(A, C) had been recovered from the bloodstain. A suspect had been apprehended who genotypically matched the crimescene blood. What would be the value of this evidence?

Ülküer *et al.* (1999) published the genotype frequencies for a Turkish population which appear in Table 14.1. From Equation 27 in Chapter 9 (p. 114) the value of evidence is given by the likelihood ratio:

$$LR = \frac{\Pr(E \mid \text{H}_\text{P})}{\Pr(E \mid \text{H}_\text{d})}$$

where E is the evidence and H_P and H_d are the propositions. The proposition H_P in this case is that the bloodstain has its origin in the suspect, that is, the suspect left the bloodstain. H_d is that the bloodstain came from someone other than the suspect. If the bloodstain came from the suspect one would expect to see the bloodstain with the same genetic profile as the suspect with probability of 1, that is, were the bloodstain to have come from the suspect it could have no other profile.

If the bloodstain originated in someone other than the suspect we could expect the evidence to be observed with a probability of the frequency of the particular combination of genotypes for LDLR, GYPA, HBGG, D7S8 and Gc. If there is independence between loci then the relative frequency of the whole profile in the population is the product of the relative frequencies of the genotypes. From Table 14.1 this is $0.127 \times 0.522 \times 0.306 \times 0.522 \times 0.159 = 0.00168$, so the value of the evidence is ≈ 594. That is, the profile is 594 times as likely to be observed were the crimescene profile to have come from the suspect than were it to have come from any other individual in the population.

The assumption has been made above that there is independence between loci. This is called *linkage equilibrium*, which is the notion that the alleles appearing on

Table 14.1 Genotype frequencies for LDLR, GYPA, HBGG, D7S8 and Gc in a sample from a Turkish population from Ülküer *et al.* (1999). Reproduced with permission

Locus	Genotype	Observed	Frequency
LDLR	*A A*	20	0.127
	A B	79	0.503
	B B	58	0.370
GYPA	*A A*	48	0.306
	A B	82	0.522
	B B	27	0.172
HBGG	*A A*	18	0.115
	A B	90	0.573
	B B	48	0.306
	A C	1	0.006
	B C	0	0.000
	C C	0	0.000
D7S8	*A A*	60	0.382
	A B	82	0.522
	B B	15	0.096
Gc	*A A*	10	0.064
	A B	13	0.083
	B B	7	0.045
	A C	48	0.306
	B C	25	0.159
	C C	54	0.343

one locus are independent of the alleles appearing on any other locus. For instance, the genotype LDLR(A, A) does not mean that GYPA is more likely to be (A, B) than any other possible GYPA genotype.

The power of DNA is that for a complete sequence of genotypes from a population there will only be a small number of people who will share that same information. However, this is also a problem with DNA because it would be extremely hard work, not to mention illegal in most jurisdictions, to sequence the entire population and store that in some databank. If all DNA profiles were known then it would be a simple matter to see how many matched a crime scene profile and a value of evidence calculated accordingly. However, this is not currently possible and much of the seeming complexity of DNA evidence is directed towards making suitable approximations in the face of incomplete evidence.

Most of the reports listing DNA in various populations in the *Journal of Forensic Sciences* report the relative frequencies of the alleles rather than the genotypes for the loci. What allows the reporting and subsequent calculation of genotype frequencies from alleic frequencies is another independence principle, that of *Hardy-Weinberg equilibrium*, which is the idea that each allele on a locus appears independently of each other allele on that locus, that is, that one allele, say, A, on the LDLR locus is no more likely to be paired with any other particular allele.

14.3 Hardy-Weinberg equilibrium

Underlying Hardy-Weinberg equilibrium is the assumption of an infinite population and random mating. These are not true, and indeed cannot be true in any absolute sense, but are approximations which, with some exceptions, are good enough for forensic purposes.

The system from Ülküer *et al.* (1999) in Table 14.1 is a relatively simple system of five loci, three of which have two possible alleles, two having three possible alleles. Even in this system the locus HBGG which has possible alleles A, B and C, hence six possible genotypes, has two genotypes (BC,CC) which have not been observed. This could be because they simply do not exist in the population, or because the sample is based on only 157 individuals from the population. Genotype AC of the HBGG locus occurs once, by substituting 0.006 for γ into Equation 32 on p. ... we would have to examine a minimum of 498 individuals to stand a 0.98 probability of observing any individuals which occur with this probability. Some of the more variable loci used in forensic science can have as many as 20 alleles, giving 210 possible genotypes. If each genotype were to occur with a uniform distribution then the probability of occurrence would be $1/210 \approx 0.005$, substituting this into Equation 32 we would have to examine at least 628 individuals to obtain a 95% probability of observing each genotype.

It is this need to be able to estimate genotypic frequencies for genotypes which have not been directly observed which makes it necessary to use loci which approximate to Hardy-Weinberg equilibrium.

First we need a way of calculating the proportion of any given allele in the sample. Examining the LDLR locus in Table 14.1 we have three possible genotypes AA, AB and BB. Denote the proportion as P with subscripts referring to the allele classification, so P_{AA} means the proportion of genotype AA, P_B would mean the proportion of allele B.

The total proportion of allele A is the proportion of genotype AA, with a contribution of half that of AB, because AB has a half portion of allele A. So $P_A = P_{AA} + 1/2P_{AB} = 0.127 + (0.503/2) = 0.3785$ and $P_B = 0.370 + (0.503/2) = 0.6215$ for the LDLR locus with genotype proportions from Table 14.1.

For a locus such as Gc with three alleles, hence six genotypes: AA, AB, AC, BB, BC and CC. Again taking the genotype proportions from Table 14.1 $P_A = P_{AA} + (P_{AB} + P_{AC})/2$ which is $0.064 + (0.083 + 0.306)/2 = 0.2585$.

A general expression for the proportions of alleles from a sample of genotypes with n alleles is:

$$P_i = P_{ii} + \frac{1}{2}\sum_{i\neq j}^{n} P_{ij} \tag{33}$$

As P_i is a proportion of all $1, \ldots, n$ alleles it can be regarded as a probability of the occurrence of P_i which will be denoted Pr_i.

Above we have an expression relating allele frequencies to genotype frequencies. The next problem is to derive some way of calculating genotype frequencies from allele frequencies.

If Hardy-Weinberg equilibrium is assumed it is possible to calculate the frequencies of all genotypes amongst the offspring of all parental offspring. We shall do this for a locus such as LDLR which has only two alleles. For any set of maternal and paternal genotypes there are only four possible offspring. For instance, if the maternal genotype is AA and the paternal is also AA then the offspring can be AA, AA, AA or AA. In other words it is guaranteed the offspring of two homozygous AA parents is homozygous AA. If the maternal genotype were again AA, but this time the paternal AB then the possible offspring are: AA, AB, AA or AB. This means that half the offspring of AA and AB will be AA, and half AB. This is tabulated for the whole LDLR locus in Table 14.2.

Table 14.2 Genotype frequencies for LDLR in offspring assuming Hardy-Weinberg equilibrium

Parental			Offspring		
Maternal	Paternal	Probability	AA	AB	BB
AA	AA	$\text{Pr}_{AA} \times \text{Pr}_{AA}$	1	0	0
	AB	$\text{Pr}_{AA} \times \text{Pr}_{AB}$	1/2	1/2	0
	BB	$\text{Pr}_{AA} \times \text{Pr}_{BB}$	0	1	0
AB	AA	$\text{Pr}_{AB} \times \text{Pr}_{AA}$	1/2	1/2	0
	AB	$\text{Pr}_{AB} \times \text{Pr}_{AB}$	1/4	1/2	1/4
	BB	$\text{Pr}_{AB} \times \text{Pr}_{BB}$	0	1/2	1/2
BB	AA	$\text{Pr}_{BB} \times \text{Pr}_{AA}$	0	1	0
	AB	$\text{Pr}_{BB} \times \text{Pr}_{AB}$	0	1/2	1/2
	BB	$\text{Pr}_{BB} \times \text{Pr}_{BB}$	0	0	1/2

Calculating the probability of seeing an AA homozygote amongst the children we can simply add the probabilities for AA from rows 1, 2, 4 and 5 in Table 14.2 which is:

$$\text{Pr}_{AA} = \text{Pr}_{AA}\text{Pr}_{AA} + \frac{1}{2}(\text{Pr}_{AA}\text{Pr}_{AB}) + \frac{1}{2}(\text{Pr}_{AB}\text{Pr}_{AA}) + \frac{1}{4}(\text{Pr}_{AB}\text{Pr}_{AB})$$

$$= \left[\text{Pr}_{AA} + \frac{1}{2}(\text{Pr}_{AB})\right]^2$$

Referring to Equation 33:

$$\text{Pr}_{AA} = \text{Pr}_A{}^2$$

For heterozygote offspring we use rows $2, 3, 4, 5, 6, 7$ and 8 from column 2 in Table 14.2.

$$\text{Pr}_{AB} = \frac{1}{2}(\text{Pr}_{AA}\text{Pr}_{AB}) + \text{Pr}_{AA}\text{Pr}_{BB} + \frac{1}{2}(\text{Pr}_{AB}\text{Pr}_{AA}) + \frac{1}{2}(\text{Pr}_{AB}\text{Pr}_{AB})$$

$$+ \frac{1}{2}(\text{Pr}_{AB}\text{Pr}_{BB}) + \text{Pr}_{BB}\text{Pr}_{AA} + \frac{1}{2}(\text{Pr}_{BB}\text{Pr}_{AB})$$

$$= 2\left[\text{Pr}_{AA} + \frac{1}{2}(\text{Pr}_{AB})\right]\left[\text{Pr}_{BB} + \frac{1}{2}(\text{Pr}_{AB})\right]$$

$$= 2\text{Pr}_A\text{Pr}_B$$

If the same calculations are made for the offspring of the offspring it is found that they are in the same proportions as the offspring. The system is now said to be in equilibrium. In general, for an unspecified number of alleles the Hardy-Weinberg law is:

$$\left.\begin{array}{l}\text{Pr}_{ii} = \text{Pr}_i^2 \\ \text{Pr}_{ij} = 2\,\text{Pr}_i\,\text{Pr}_j, \quad j \neq i\end{array}\right\} \tag{34}$$

Using Equation 34 it is now possible to calculate possible frequencies for the genotypes BC and CC on the HBGG locus. HBGG has three alleles A, B and C. The proportion of A alleles can be calculated by $P_A = P_{AA} + \frac{1}{2}(P_{AB} + P_{AC})$ which is $0.115 + \frac{1}{2}(0.573 + 0.006) = 0.4045$. Likewise P_B can be shown to be 0.5925 and $P_C = 0.003$.

BC is heterozygous, thus from Equation 34 $\text{Pr}_{BC} = 2\,\text{Pr}_B\,\text{Pr}_C$ which evaluates to $\text{Pr}_{BC} = 2 \times 0.5925 \times 0.003 = 0.0035$, CC being homozygous $\text{Pr}_{CC} = \text{Pr}_C{}^2$ which occurs with probability $0.003^2 = 0.000009$.

At this stage it should be pointed out that Ülküer *et al.* (1999) state that Hardy-Weinberg equilibrium was found not to be the case for locus HBGG from their Turkish population, and that they could find no reason why this should be the case in their investigations. Testing for Hardy-Weinberg equilibrium is a whole topic in its own right and will not be pursued further here.

14.4 Simple case allelic frequencies

Returning to the example in Section 14.2, suppose blood had been recovered from broken glass at a crimescene in Turkey. The genotypes TPOX(6, 9), VWA(17, 17) and TH01(9, 9.3) had been identified from this. A suspect had been apprehended who genotypically matched the crimescene blood. What would be the value of this evidence?

From Equation 27 in Chapter 9 (p. 114) the value of evidence is given by the likelihood ratio:

$$\text{LR} = \frac{\text{Pr}(E \mid \text{H}_\text{P})}{\text{Pr}(E \mid \text{H}_\text{d})}$$

where E is the evidence and H_P and H_d are the propositions. The proposition H_P in this case is that the profile observed in the bloodstain came from the suspect. H_d is that the profile observed from the bloodstain came from someone other than the suspect. If the bloodstain came from the suspect one would expect to see the bloodstain with the same genetic profile as the suspect with probability of 1, that is, were the bloodstain to have come from the suspect it could have no other profile.

If the bloodstain originated in someone other than the suspect we could expect the evidence to be observed with a probability of the frequency of the particular combination of genotypes for TPOX, VWA, and THO1.

Çakir et al. (2001) give the allelic frequencies (see Table 14.3) for individuals convicted of a criminal offence in Turkey.

Table 14.3 Allele frequencies for TPOX, VWA and THO1 in Turkey, from Çakir et al. (2001). Reproduced with permission

Locus	Allele	Relative Frequency
TPOX	6	0.006
	8	0.506
	9	0.094
	10	0.063
	11	0.294
	12	0.038
VWA	14	0.086
	15	0.067
	16	0.276
	17	0.300
	18	0.205
	19	0.048
	20	0.001
	21	0.001
THO1	6	0.295
	7	0.147
	8	0.184
	9	0.232
	9.3	0.026
	10	0.116

To calculate the frequency for the observed profile assuming both Hardy-Weinberg and linkage equilibria we observe that the TPOX locus from the bloodstain has alleles 6 and 9. Allele 6 occurs with a frequency of 0.006 and 9 with a relative frequency 0.094. Substituting these values into Equation 34 for heterozygosity the frequency of TPOX(6, 9) is $2 \times 0.006 \times 0.094 = 0.001128$. For the homozygosity at VWA(17, 17) the frequency is $0.30^2 = 0.09$. Allele 9 on the THO1 locus occurs with a frequency 0.232, and allele 9.3 with 0.026, so THO1(9, 9.3) occurs

$2 \times 0.232 \times 0.026 = 0.012064$. As linkage equilibrium has been assumed the frequency of the observed profile is $0.001128 \times 0.09 \times 0.012064 = 1.224737 \times 10^{-6}$ hence the evidential value is $1/1.224737 \times 10^{-6} = 816501$. That is, the observation of that particular profile is 816501 times as likely were the bloodstain to have come from the suspect than from anyone else in the Turkish population.

14.5 Accounting for sub-populations

In Section 14.3 we looked at a simple case assuming Hardy-Weinberg equilibrium. We said that the conditions for Hardy-Weinberg equilibrium were seldom met, in fact could not in principle be fully met, but that it was a good initial starting position. Here we examine the more realistic case where the population under consideration comprises various sub-populations caused by the fact that mating has not been uniformly random throughout the whole population in previous generations. This could be caused by geographic proximity, for example individuals in Cornwall are far more likely to mate with those in the South-West of England, than with individuals in North-West Scotland, or they may be social, where people of different ethnic origins will tend to reproduce within their own ethnic grouping.

Evett and Weir (1998, p. 107) give the following for the probabilities of individuals from a sub-population receiving alleles A_i and A_j given the populational relative frequencies p_i and p_j with a co-ancestry coefficient F which is the probability of two alleles drawn from the same sub-population being identical through descent:

$$\left. \begin{array}{l} \mathrm{Pr}_{ii} = p_i^2 + p_i(1 - p_i)F \\ \mathrm{Pr}_{ij} = 2p_i p_j(1 - F) \end{array} \right\}$$

They then show how these lead to the expressions given by Balding and Nichols (1997):

$$\left. \begin{array}{l} \mathrm{Pr}_{ii} = \dfrac{[2F + (1 - F)p_i][3F + (1 - F)p_i]}{(1 + F)(1 + 2F)} \\[4mm] \mathrm{Pr}_{ij} = \dfrac{2[F + (1 - F)p_i][F + (1 - F)p_j]}{(1 + F)(1 + 2F)} \end{array} \right\} \tag{35}$$

where $i \neq j$.

Equation 35 is a direct replacement for Equation 34 on page .... Note, if F in Equation 35 is equal to zero, then Equation 35 will evaluate to Equation 34, so Equation 34 can be seen as a special case of Equation 35 with $F = 0$.

The problem with Equation 35 is the extra parameter F, or the co-ancestry coefficient. Evett and Weir (1998, p. 159) discuss no fewer than three different measures of sub-population inbreeding:

- *within-population inbreeding coefficient* f' – the extent to which two alleles are related compared with pairs of alleles in different individuals in the same sub-population.

- *total inbreeding coefficient f* – extent of relatedness of alleles within an individual compared with alleles in the whole population.

- *coancestry coefficient F* – the relatedness between alleles of different individuals in one sub-population compared with other sub-populations.

which are related by:

$$f = \frac{f' - F}{1 - F}$$

To evaluate (35) we are only interested in the *coancestry coefficient* [†].

If ϕ_1 is the mean square of the proportion of allele i among sub-populations, and ϕ is the mean square of the proportion of allele i between sub-populations, these are evaluated:

$$\phi_1 = \frac{2n}{r - 1} \sum_{s=1}^{r} (\hat{p}_{is} - \overline{p}_i)^2$$

$$\phi = \frac{2n}{r(2n - 1)} \sum_{s=1}^{r} \hat{p}_{is}(1 - \hat{p}_{is})$$

where there are r sub-populations, n genotypes, the relative frequency of allele i being estimates as $\hat{p}_{is}$ for each sub-population, and $\overline{p}_i$ is the mean of r $\hat{p}_{is}$.

An estimate of F can be made by (Evett and Weir, 1998, p. 161):

$$\frac{\phi_1 - \phi}{\phi_1 + (2n - 1)\phi} = \frac{F_w - F}{1 - F}$$

where F_w is the mean of all the F's that apply to each of the r sub-populations.

Technically there should be a specific value of F for each and every combination of alleles at the locus, however, it is simply not possible to produce a definitive list of sub-populations for any natural population. As a large value of F favours the defence it has been practice to select a value towards the upper end of those values of F which have been calculated. Currently the recommendation is $F = 0.03$ (NRC, 1996).

For example, earlier we observed the TPOX locus with alleles 6 and 9, VWA(17, 17) and THO1(9, 9.3) in a Turkish population. Taking alleic frequencies from Table 14.3, and $F = 0.03$, substituting into Equation 35 the genotypic frequencies for TPOX(6, 9) is 0.0079, VWA(17, 17) is 0.1225 and THO1(9, 9.3) is 0.0258. Assuming linkage equilibrium the product of these is 2.50×10^{-5} which yields a value of 40,0051 rather than the 816501 calculated in Section 14.4, and is a considerable reduction in the value of the observed evidence.

[†] Denoted by F here, and θ in Evett and Weir (1998).

Review questions

1. Use Table 14.1 to calculate the alleic frequencies for LDLR(A) GYPA(A) and GYPA(B), HBGG(B), D758(A) and D788(B) and Gc(A) and Gc(B). Assume Hardy-Weinburg equllibrian and linkage equllibriam to calculate an evidential value of a match in an uncomplicated case where 60th the suspect and offender are LDLR(A,A) GYPA(A,B); HBGG(B,B), D758(A,B) and Gc(A,C).

2. Compare it with the value listed calculated directly from the genotype frequencies listed in Table 14.1.

3. Why might these be different?

4. Calculate the value of the profile above without assuming Hardy-Weinberg equilibrium. The co-ancestry coefficient can be assumed to be 0.03.

15

DNA II

This chapter addresses the question of the evaluation of DNA evidence in paternity (or maternity) assignment, and some of the current debates in forensic DNA such as the *database search* problem.

15.1 Paternity – mother and father unrelated

One of the areas in civil law where forensic science is extensively employed is the DNA testing for paternity. Typically these cases will consist of a mother who claims a specific individual is the father of her offspring. A DNA profile will have been collected from the child, the mother and the putative father. Usually, from any single locus, the evidence E will comprise: G_c the child's genotype, G_m the maternal genotype, G_{pp} the putative paternal genotype. Let G_p be the true paternal genotype.

For the locus under consideration G_c will have two alleles, A_m from maternal inheritance, and A_p from paternal inheritance.

The questions under consideration are whether G_c could have been the offspring of G_m and G_{pp}, and, if so, what would be the value of the DNA evidence?

Obviously some combinations of G_{pp}, G_c will exclude the proposition $G_{pp} = G_p$, for instance were $G_c(i, \ j)$, $G_m(i, \ k)$ and $G_{pp}(k, \ l)$ then $G_{pp} \neq G_p$ as there are no common alleles between putative father and offspring[†].

Denote two propositions:

$$H_p \equiv G_{pp} = G_p$$

$$H_d \equiv G_{pp} \neq G_p$$

[†] In this case we can go further in saying that A_i must have been maternally inherited, therefore at least one of the paternal alleles must be A_j.

Introduction to Statistics for Forensic Scientists   David Lucy
© 2005 John Wiley & Sons, Ltd.

Evett and Weir (1998, p. 165) give the following expression for a likelikhood ratio:

$$LR = \frac{\Pr(G_c \mid G_m, G_{pp}, H_p)}{\Pr(G_c \mid G_m, G_{pp}, H_d)} \tag{36}$$

where background information I has been omitted for clarity. Equation 36 is the probability of observing the offspring's genotype given the maternal genotype, the putative paternal genotype and two propositions; and is a version of Equation 27 in Section 9.3 on p. 114.

If the numerator of Equation 36 is examined:

$$\text{numerator} = \Pr(G_c \mid G_m, G_{pp}, H_p)$$

$$= \Pr(A_m, \ A_p \mid G_m, G_{pp}, H_p)$$

$$= \Pr(A_m \mid G_m, G_{pp}, H_p)\Pr(A_p \mid A_m, G_m, G_{pp}, H_p)$$

As A_m depends solely on G_m, and A_p upon G_p, and under H_p $G_{pp} = G_p$ then:

$$\Pr(A_m \mid G_m, G_{pp}, H_p) = \Pr(A_m \mid G_m)$$

$$\Pr(A_p \mid A_m G_m, G_{pp}, H_p = \Pr(A_p \mid G_{pp}, H_p)$$

so:

$$\text{numerator} = \Pr(A_m \mid G_m) \, \Pr(A_p \mid G_{pp}, H_p) \tag{37}$$

which is a general expression for the numerator.

Applying Equation 37 to the case where G_c is homozygous ($G_c = (A_i, \ A_i)$) the numerator is:

$$\text{numerator} = \Pr(A_m = A_i \mid G_m) \, \Pr(A_p = A_i \mid G_{pp}, \ H_p)$$

For example, were $G_c(i, \ i)$, $G_m(i, \ j)$ and $G_{pp}(i, \ k)$ the probability of $A_m = A_i$ is 1/2 as there is only one way in which A_i could have been passed down, but either A_i or A_j could have been inherited. A similar argument applied to $A_p = A_i$ as the true father passed down A_i, and the putative paternal genotype could have passed either A_i or A_k; hence $\Pr(A_p = A_i \mid G_{pp}, \ H_p = 1/2)$ so the numerator is $1/2 \times 1/2 = 1/4$.

Where the offspring is heterozygous matters are a little more complicated as we have no information about which allele came from which parent, so if $G_c(i, \ j)$ then:

$$\text{numerator} = \Pr(A_m = A_i \mid G_m) \, \Pr(A_p = A_j \mid G_{pp}, \ H_p)$$

$$+ \Pr(A_m = A_j \mid G_m) \, \Pr(A_p = A_i \mid G_{pp}, \ H_p)$$

For example, given $G_c(i, \ j)$, $G_m(i, \ j)$ and $G_{pp}(j, \ k)$:

$$\Pr(A_m = A_i \mid G_m) = 1/2$$

$$\Pr(A_p = A_j \mid G_{pp}, \ H_p) = 1/2$$

$$\Pr(A_m = A_j \mid G_m) = 1/2$$

$$\Pr(A_p = A_i \mid G_{pp}, \ H_p) = 0$$

The numerator in this case would be $(1/2 \times 1/2) + (1/2 \times 0) = 1/4$.

Evett and Weir (1998, p. 167) use a similar line of reasoning for the denominator for Equation 36 which they give as:

$$\text{denominator} = \Pr(A_m \mid G_m, H_d) \, \Pr(A_p \mid A_m, G_m, G_{pp}, H_d)$$

which as the proposition this time is $H_d \equiv G_{pp} \neq G_p$, A_p is not dependent on G_{pp}. So, as for the numerator:

$$\text{denominator} = \Pr(A_m \mid G_m) \Pr(A_p \mid H_d)$$

$$\text{homozygous offspring} = \Pr(A_m = A_i \mid G_m) \Pr(A_p = A_i \mid H_d)$$

$$\text{heterozygous offspring} = \Pr(A_m = A_i \mid G_m) \Pr(A_p = A_j \mid H_d)$$
$$+ \Pr(A_m = A_j \mid G_m) \Pr(A_p = A_i \mid H_d)$$

For instance, were $G_c(i, i)$, $G_m(i, j)$ and $G_{pp}(i, i)$, then $\Pr(A_m = A_i \mid G_m) = 1/2$ as the maternal genotype shares a single allele with the offspring. The paternal allele $A_p = A_i$ which occurs with relative frequency p_i in the relevant population, so $\Pr(A_p = A_i \mid H_d) = p_i$ which makes the denominator $p_i/2$.

Were $G_c(i, j)$, $G_m(i, k)$ and $G_{pp}(j, j)$ then $\Pr(A_m = A_i \mid G_m) = 1/2$, $\Pr(A_m = A_j \mid G_m) = 0$, $\Pr(A_p = A_i \mid H_d) = p_i$ and $\Pr(A_p = A_j \mid H_d) = p_j$; making the denominator $\frac{1}{2}p_j + 0 p_i = \frac{1}{2}p_j$.

Possible combinations of offspring, maternal genotype and paternal genotype are given in Table 15.1. This can be used as a simple lookup table.

Suppose a paternity case came about in Turkey where a woman claimed that a specific man was the father of the child. Profiles were obtained for TPOX, VWA and THO1 for offspring, maternal and putative paternal. These are given in Table 15.2.

Taking the TPOX locus first, and let allele $6 = i$, $9 = j$, $12 = k$ and $l = 8$. This makes $G_c(i, j)$, $G_m(i, k)$ and $G_{pp}(j, l)$. Referring to the second from bottom line in Table 15.1 that genotype combination has a numerator of $1/4$ and a denominator of $p_j/2$ thus a likelihood ratio of $1/(2p_j)$. p_j in this case is the TPOX allele 9 which from Table 14.3 has a relative frequency of 0.094 in the Turkish population, so the likelihood ratio associated with this is 5.32.

Next consider the VWA locus. Let allele $17 = i$ and $16 = j$. $G_c(i, i)$, $G_m(i, j)$ and $G_{pp}(i, i)$. This corresponds to the fourth row of Table 15.1 where the numerator is $1/2$, the denominator $pi/2$, hence likelihood ratio $1/pi$. i is allele 17 in the Turkish population, and from Table 14.3 has a relative frequency of 0.3 making the likelihood ratio 3.33.

Finally the THO1 locus. Let allele $9 = i$, $7 = j$, and $10 = k$. The genotypes can then be said to be $G_o(i, j)$, $G_m(i, k)$ and $G_{pp}(i, j)$. This is given in Table 15.1 on the fourth row from bottom. The numerator is $1/4$, the denominator $p_j/2$, the likelihood ratio $1/(2p_j)$. Allele j is 7 which occurs with relative frequency 0.147 from Table 14.3, the corresponding likelihood ratio being 3.40.

Assuming linkage equilibrium the value for all the profiles is $5.32 \times 3.33 \times 3.4 = 60.23$ which means that these profiles are ≈ 60 times more likely were the putative paternal profile the true paternal profile of G_c in the Turkish population.

Table 15.1 Numerator, denominator and likelihood ratios in paternity testing. Recalculated from Evett and Weir (1998). Reproduced with permission

G_c	G_m	G_{pp}	numerator	denominator	LR
$A_i\,A_i$	$A_i\,A_i$	$A_i\,A_i$	1	p_i	$\frac{1}{p_i}$
		$A_i\,A_j$	$\frac{1}{2}$	p_i	$\frac{1}{2p_i}$
		$A_j\,A_k$	0	p_i	0
	$A_i\,A_j$	$A_i\,A_i$	$\frac{1}{2}$	$\frac{p_i}{2}$	$\frac{1}{p_i}$
		$A_i\,A_j$	$\frac{1}{4}$	$\frac{p_i}{2}$	$\frac{1}{2p_i}$
		$A_i\,A_k$	$\frac{1}{4}$	$\frac{p_i}{2}$	$\frac{1}{2p_i}$
		$A_j\,A_k$	0	$\frac{p_i}{2}$	0
$A_i\,A_j$	$A_i\,A_i$	$A_j\,A_j$	1	p_j	$\frac{1}{p_j}$
		$A_i\,A_j$	$\frac{1}{2}$	p_j	$\frac{1}{2p_j}$
		$A_j\,A_k$	$\frac{1}{2}$	p_j	$\frac{1}{2p_j}$
		$A_k\,A_l$	0	p_j	0
	$A_i\,A_j$	$A_i\,A_i$	$\frac{1}{2}$	$\frac{p_i+p_j}{2}$	$\frac{1}{p_i+p_j}$
		$A_i\,A_j$	$\frac{1}{2}$	$\frac{p_i+p_j}{2}$	$\frac{1}{p_i+p_j}$
		$A_i\,A_k$	$\frac{1}{4}$	$\frac{p_i+p_j}{2}$	$\frac{1}{2(p_i+p_j)}$
		$A_j\,A_k$	$\frac{1}{4}$	$\frac{p_i+p_j}{2}$	$\frac{1}{2(p_i+p_j)}$
		$A_k\,A_l$	0	$\frac{p_i+p_j}{2}$	0
	$A_i\,A_k$	$A_j\,A_j$	$\frac{1}{2}$	$\frac{p_j}{2}$	$\frac{1}{p_j}$
		$A_i\,A_j$	$\frac{1}{4}$	$\frac{p_j}{2}$	$\frac{1}{2p_j}$
		$A_j\,A_k$	$\frac{1}{4}$	$\frac{p_j}{2}$	$\frac{1}{2p_j}$
		$A_j\,A_l$	$\frac{1}{4}$	$\frac{p_j}{2}$	$\frac{1}{2p_j}$
		$A_k\,A_l$	0	$\frac{p_j}{2}$	0

Table 15.2 Genotypes (simulated) from a paternity example from Turkey

locus	G_c	G_m	G_{pp}
TPOX	(6, 9)	(6, 12)	(8, 9)
VWA	(17, 17)	(17, 16)	(17, 17)
THO1	(7, 9)	(9, 10)	(7, 9)

15.2 Database searches and value of evidence

The question of the value of a match from a DNA database search has been a vexed one, but as the database of profiles in the United Kingdom now[‡] numbers 2.1 million profiles, it is increasingly and relevant one.

[‡] January 2005.

The essential dispute revolves around the question of whether the evidential value is higher if a suspect is selected from a database of n individuals as $n - 1$ individuals have been excluded, or is the evidential value lower because there has been potentially n goes at getting a match.

The National Research Council (1996) argument runs along the latter lines. For the situation where a DNA profile at a crimescene (E_c) matches that of a suspect (E_s) located from a DNA database search:

- *prosecution case H_p* – E_c matches that of E_s because the suspect is the source of the crimescene DNA.

- *defence case H_d* – the match between E_c and E_s is entirely coincidental, the suspect is not the source of the crimescene DNA.

From Equation 9.5 on p. .... the value of the evidence is given by:

$$V = \frac{Pr(E_c = E_s \mid H_p, I)}{Pr(E_c \equiv E_s \mid H_d, I)}$$

where I is background information. In the simplest case if H_p is true then $Pr(E_c = E_s \mid H_p, I) = 1$, so:

$$V = \frac{1}{Pr(E_c \equiv E_s \mid H_d, I)} = \frac{1}{p}$$

If the DNA profile at the crimescene occurs with probability p in the population, and, there are n randomly selected unrelated individuals in the database, then the probability that any individual from the population does not match the crimescene profile is $1 - p$, assuming independence the probability no individuals from the database match the crimescene is $(1 - p)^n$. Therefore the probability at least one profile from the database matches is $1 - (1 - p)^n$, which for small p, $\approx np$. So according to the National Research Council (1996) $V = 1/np$ in the simplest case.

This position was re-enforced by Stockmarr (1999) who derived the same result and contradicted other workers in the field such as Balding and Donnelly (1995) and Evett and Weir (1998). Eventually the debate resulted in a rather acrimonious series of letters in the journal *Biometrics* (Evett and Foreman, 2000; Devlin, 2000).

Balding and Donnelly (1995) took a different view to the National Research Council (1996) and Stockmarr (1999). Their work first examines the case where a genetic profile is found at a crimescene, a suspect is identified, a genetic profile observed, and it is found to match that at the crimescene. This they termed the *probable cause* argument. Balding and Donnelly (1995) consider this single individual as a database of 1, and expand their consideration to databases of size n with roughly the same result that the value is $\approx 1/p$ where p is the probability of occurrence of the genetic profile in the population.

The problem is that n is a sample from a larger population N. As the database grows larger, and n approaches N, **V** grows smaller. In the case where $n = N$ and everybody in the population is represented in the database the DNA evidence is at its minimum value, whereas intuition would suggest it is at its maximum value because all other possibilities have been excluded.

Evett and Foreman (2000) argue Stockmarr (1999) calculated the ratio of the probabilities for the propositions:

- *prosecution hypothesis* – one of the individuals in the database left the crime stain

- *defence hypothesis* – some person other than the n individuals in the database left the crime scene

which they claimed gave a posterior probability ratio rather than:

- *prosecution hypothesis* – the suspect left the crimescene profile

- *defence hypothesis* – some person other than the suspect left the profile at the crimescene

which if the likelihood ratio is calculated using the latter hypothesis then the correct likelihood ratio is obtained.

15.3 Discussion

The discussion over database searching is likely to continue for some time with most researchers in the field being in the $1/p$ group (Dawid, 2001), and a minority in the $1/np$ group. The current[§] advice in the United Kingdom is to follow the advice of Evett & Weir (1998) and others in the $1/p$ group.

Future developments are going to include ways of managing weights of evidence under non-equilibrium conditions. We have already seen in Section 14.5 how to do this under conditions where Hardy-Weinberg equilibrium may not hold. Buckleton *et al.* (2001) discuss how failure to find deviations from linkage and Hardy-Weinberg equilibrium does not necessarily mean independence can be assumed. The answer may be to develop methods which can operate from allelic frequencies, but do not require independence.

[§] January 2005.

Review questions

1. Suppose a woman in Turkey claims paternity against a Turkish man whose DNA profiles are measured and the data in the following table is produced:

locus	G_c	G_m	G_{pp}
TPOX	(6, 6)	(9, 6)	(12, 6)
VWA	(18, 21)	(16, 21)	(18, 21)
THO1	(9, 9.3)	(6, 9.3)	(9, 10)

Assuming Hardy-Weinberg and linkage equilibrium apply, what is the value of this evidence in favour of the proposition $G_{pp} = G_p$?

2. Suppose a woman in Turkey claims paternity against a Turkish man whose DNA profiles are measured and the data in the following table produced:

locus	G_c	G_m	G_{pp}
TPOX	(6, 6)	(9, 6)	(12, 6)
VWA	(18, 21)	(16, 21)	(18, 21)
THO1	(9, 9.3)	(6, 9.3)	(8, 10)

Assuming Hardy-Weinberg and linkage equilibrium apply what is the value of this evidence in favour of the proposition $G_{pp} = G_p$?

3. Suppose a woman in Turkey claims paternity against a Turkish man. DNA profiles are measured and the data in the following table are produced:

locus	G_c	G_m	G_{pp}
LDLR	(A, B)	(A, B)	(B, B)
GYPA	(A, B)	(A, A)	(B, B)
HBGG	(B, B)	(B, B)	(B, B)
D7S8	(A, B)	(A, B)	(A, B)
Gc	(A, C)	(A, B)	(B, C)

Assuming Hardy-Weinberg and linkage equilibrium apply what is the value of this evidence in favour of the proposition $G_{pp} = G_p$?

16 Sampling and sample size estimation

For the forensic scientist sample size estimation is one of the trickier areas of statistics. However, for laboratory based forensic scientists it is important to have some well-founded idea of a relevant sample size. This is because the results, and hence the conclusions, from an experiment based upon too few observations are not going to be in the least reliable, and from the point of view of forensic practice, and experiment which is 'over-sampled' is wasteful of resources.

The reason sample size estimation is tricky is not because the mathematical parts are particularly complex, but because the amount of information which needs to be known is large, and cannot necessarily be known with any precision before the beginning of an experiment. This entails that a large number of unformed 'guesses' and approximations usually have to be made, and that the resultant sample size estimate made prior to an experiment is more of a guide to how large a sample should be taken, rather than any exact number. This does not make these estimates worthless, or pointless, for they are still very useful in that it is better to have some idea of the order of the sample size, for example whether one needs to sample 10s or 100s, than no idea whatsoever.

16.1 Estimation of a mean

In Sections 4.2 and 4.4 we saw that a confidence interval at some level, say $\alpha\%$, for a mean can be calculated from the sample standard deviation and knowledge of the relevant t-distribution. To recap, the standard error of the mean can be calculated from Equation 7 on p. 31, and is:

$$\text{standard error of the mean } (x) = \frac{\text{sd}}{\sqrt{n}}$$

Introduction to Statistics for Forensic Scientists   David Lucy
© 2005 John Wiley & Sons, Ltd.

sd being the sample standard deviation. To calculate the confidence interval the resultant standard error of the mean is multiplied by the ordinate of the αth point on the t-distribution with $n - 1$ degrees of freedom.

If we wish to go the other way, and find out what would be an appropriate value of n to obtain a confidence interval of some predefined magnitude at some predefined level of confidence?

The problem here is to enable us to select the correct t-distribution we need to know what n is, and n is the value we are trying to calculate. A common solution (Devore and Peck, 1997) is to disregard the fact that a t-distribution gives the appropriate factor by which to multiply the standard error of the mean, and instead approximate the t with a normal.

For example, in Figure 4.4 on p. 33 we saw that, based on a sample of 20 measurements of Δ^9-THC from marijuana seizures in 1986, the mean was 8.59% THC, the standard deviation being 1.09%. How many observations would one need to ensure with a 99% confidence that the true mean was known to within $\pm 0.3\%$-THC.

From Appendix C we know that 99% of the standard normal curve is between -2.58 and 2.58 standard deviations by looking up the ordinate for the area at 0.995 (we wish to leave 0.005 in *each* tail). The interval we wish to calculate is ± 2.58 standard errors, and is 0.3%. As 0.3 is at 2.58 standard errors one standard error is at $0.3/2.58 = 0.116$. Setting the standard error of the mean to 0.116 in the equation above, we can re-arrange to find a suitable value for n:

$$0.116 = \frac{1.09}{\sqrt{n}}$$

$$0.116 \times \sqrt{n} = 1.09$$

$$\sqrt{n} = \frac{1.09}{0.116}$$

$$n = \left(\frac{1.09}{0.116}\right)^2$$

$$= 9.397^2$$

$$= 88.30$$

We must make whole numbers of observations, so this should be rounded up to 89. A sample size of 89 seizures from 1986 would be required to be able to isolate with 99% confidence the mean of the Δ^9-THC to within 0.3%-THC. Of course, with the new sample the mean is unlikely to remain at 8.59%, and the standard deviation also unlikely to stay at 1.09%. The estimate of sample size above is therefore unlikely to be able to answer the question precisely, but it does give a good approximate idea of the sampling requirement.

Notice that without having any data upon which to base estimates of variance it is simply not possible to make an estimate of a sample size. Sample sizes cannot be calculated before anything is known; some test sampleing must be made to estimate variance.

16.2 Sample sizes for *t*-tests

Sample sizes can be calculated for both one and two sample *t*-tests, although to calculate an estimate as precise as with the standard error calculations above is far more difficult, and more has to be known in advance.

The key to sample size estimation is to find a meaningful quantity which can be calculated from data which is affected in some way by the number of observations made. Summarizing from Section 4.7:

- H_0 is a hypothesis of 'no difference'.

- A Type I error is the rejection of H_0 when H_0 is true.

- α is a pre-defined probability, called a significance level, at which making a a Type I error is acceptable.

- A *p*-value is the probability of finding the observed values, or any values more extreme, given the truth of the null hypothesis.

- Confidence is the complement of significance, that is $1 - \alpha$.

- H_1 is a hypothesis of 'difference'.

- A Type II error is the error of not rejecting H_0 when H_0 is false.

- β is the probability of making a Type II error.

- $1 - \beta$ is called the *power* of a test, and can be interpreted as the probability of detecting a difference if one exists.

It is the probability β which is related to the number of observations, and which is critical to sample size estimation in *t*-testing.

Two sample *t*-test

For both one and two sample *t*-tests it turns out that the probability β is dependent on the sample size, the level of significance for the test, and the magnitude of the difference between the population means of which sample 1 and sample 2 and samples. Calculating β is in itself a complicated process, however estimating

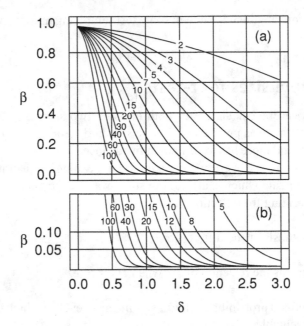

Figure 16.1 Operating characteristic curves for the two sample t-test with significance level 0.05. (a) shows the curves for all values of β. (b) shows the curves for the region $\beta \leq 0.20$

sample size can be simplified by the preparation of graphs of β against a quantity called δ for different sample sizes. These graphs are called operating characteristic curves (Montgomery, 1991), and are specific to a test. Figure 16.1 shows some of these curves for various values of n.

The quantity δ is a standardized measure of difference. In the same way that a z score is a measure of standardized distance on the standard normal curve, δ is a standardized distance between the means of the two samples. It is calculated by taking the actual magnitude of the difference between the two means you wish to detect, and dividing by twice the estimate of the standard deviation. An estimate of the standard deviation can be made by taking the square root of the estimate of pooled variance given in Equation 9 in Section 4.5. So:

$$\delta = \frac{|\text{difference}|}{2 \times \sqrt{\text{pooled variance}}}$$

where the lines $||$ in the numerator indicate the absolute value of. The values for n in Figure 16.1 are the numbers of observations in both samples. It is assumed that each sample will have roughly equal numbers in it, so the n in Figure 16.1 is in fact equal to $n_1 + n_2 - 1$. So, for example, for an n of 40 from Figure 16.1 each sample would ideally have $(40 + 1)/2 = 20.5 \approx 21$ observations in it.

It will be noticed that for the above sample size estimate we need an estimate of the variance, an estimate of the expected differences, and the significance level. There is no problem about the significance level, we select that arbitrarily. However, the expected differences and variances are more difficult to estimate. One way is to use expertise from other similar experiments to suggest suitable values for these parameters from background experience. Another way would be to perform some sort of precursor, or pilot experiment, the purpose of which is to suggest values for the sample size estimation process.

Table 4.2 on p. 39 gives the means of two samples of seized marijuana from 1985 and 1986. The mean for the 1986 sample is 8.59%; for the 1987 sample it is 7.79%. By using Equation 9 it was calculated that an estimate of the pooled variance is 0.95.%-THC.

If any future observations of 1986 and 1987 Δ^9-THC are going to have a semblance to these values which we may consider to be a pilot experiment, then we might expect to see a difference of $8.59 - 7.79 = 0.8\%$. Standardizing this we can see that we are trying to detect a difference of $0.8/(2 \times \sqrt{0.95}) = 0.41$ standardized units. So $\delta = 0.41$.

From Table 4.2 we see that $n_1 = 20$ and $n_2 = 15$, this makes n in Figure 16.1 as $20 + 15 - 1 = 34$. The nearest to 34 in Figure 16.1 is 30. Approximating 0.41 with 0.5, and following the 0.5 line up until it meets the curve for $n = 30$ in Figure 16.1, we read off from the vertical scale that β is approximately 0.55. This means that, from the previous test, there is a 55% probability that we shall make a Type II error, or say that there will be no difference in means when in fact there is one.

What value of n do we need to give us a low probability of making a Type II error? We have to pick a level for β. The two levels marked on Figure 16.1B are reasonable starting points. Let us allow a 10% probability for not rejecting H_0 when it is false. Looking along the horizontal 0.10 line on Figure 16.1B it can be observed that the 0.5 vertical line intersects somewhere between the curve for $n = 60$ and $n = 100$, and much closer to the $n = 100$ line than the $n = 60$ line. Therefore $n = 100$ will easily be an adequate estimate of the sampling requirement for this experiment.

Using Figure 16.1 is not a very precise way of estimating β for a given n, δ and α, and better results can be obtained using the precise formulae for β, however the calculations are difficult, and if a more precise estimate is required a function from some statistical software might be best employed.

One sample *t*-test

The same sort of sample size estimation can be applied to a paired *t*-test as to the two-sample *t*-test. An estimate of some expected difference δ is required, and a set of operating characteristic curves consulted to find a relevant sample size for a given β.

Taking our haploid cell example from p. 41, the observed difference from our sample is an appropriate estimate of the difference we are interested in examining, we have a mean difference of 714 cells between PBS and water extraction, and a variance of 2296438. Our value for δ is therefore:

$$\delta = \frac{\text{difference}}{2 \times \sqrt{\text{variance}}} = \frac{714}{2 \times 1515.4} = 0.23$$

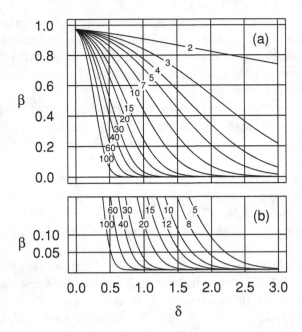

Figure 16.2 Operating characteristic curves for the one sample t-test with significance level 0.05. (a) shows the curves for all values of β. (b) shows the curves for the region $\beta \leq 0.20$

which is a very small value for δ. Consulting Figure 16.2B we find that at $\beta = 0.05$, n would have to exceed 100 pairs of observations for a $\delta = 0.5$, so $\delta = 0.23$ would require yet more pairs of observations. Again for a more precise estimate a suitable computer function should be employed.

16.3 How many drugs to sample

Over half (Nelson, *pers. comm.* 2003) of all the work undertaken by the Lothian and Borders Police Forensic Science Laboratory is related to illegal drugs. This proportion is even greater in some of the other Scottish forensic science laboratories. A major part of that work is the assessment of consignment of supposed illegal substances to find out how much of the illicit substance is contained in the seizure.

Where chemical assays are expensive, and many thousands of units may be involved, assaying all units might be prohibitively expensive. Therefore, some method of selecting a certain number of units to assay directly are needed. Sample size estimate procedures are reviewed in Izenman (2001). They include the 10% rule, where 10% of the consignment is subject to detailed examination, and the square root rule, where, in a seized consignment there are n units, then $\sqrt{n}$ units come under further scrutiny. The problem with these sample sizes is that they have no statistical basis whatsoever.

The ENFSI[†] (2003) report recommends that sample sizes be based in some way upon the statistical properties of the sample, not some arbitrary rule as described above. The reasons for this recommendation are that the set proportion (10%, $\sqrt{n}$ result in large sample sizes, and cannot lead to further inferences about the nature of the consignment based on the sample.

The Drugs Working Group of ENFSI details several methods for making inferences about a consignment from observations from a sample drawn randomly from the consignment. These inferences can be based upon a hypergeometric distribution, a binomial distribution, or beta distributions. Methods based on the beta distribution are particularly useful for large consignment (≥ 50 units) sizes, and have a further interest in that they have a far wider application field that drug consignment estimation.

Aitken (1999) employed beta distributions for a Bayesian method which, given a prior distribution for the proportion of illicit units in the consignment, data generated by observations from the consignment, and Bayes' theorem, produced a posterior density function for the proportion of illegal units in the consignment. This whole method is termed *beta-beta* the first *beta* denoting the beta used to describe the prior distribution, the second *beta* being the posterior distribution. These two distributions are combined by using a binomial likelihood.

The beta can take on several different shapes and has the property that the entire distribution is contained in the interval $0 \leq \theta \leq 1$, which makes it ideal for describing proportions. It has two parameters, α and β, which control the shape of the distribution. These can be viewed in some respects like the parameters of the normal distribution, the mean and standard deviation, but do not operate in the same way, and are not as easily interpretable as the parameters of the normal distribution.

The density at any point $0 \leq \theta \leq 1$ is given by:

$$f(\theta \mid \alpha, \beta) = \frac{\theta^{\alpha-1}(1-\theta)^{\beta-1}}{\mathbf{B}(\alpha, \beta)}$$

where:

$$\mathbf{B}(\alpha, \beta) = \frac{\Gamma(\alpha)\Gamma(\beta)}{\Gamma(\alpha + \beta)}$$

and Γ[‡] is a standard function, which for integer parameters $\Gamma(n) = (n-1)!$. Figure 16.3 shows four beta distributions with different α and β parameters.

By adjusting α and β we can set up any sort of prior distribution, from a peak over the place where we have reason to believe the true proportion of units containing drugs belongs, to a U shaped distribution which could be used to represent a prior opinion that the units in the consignment are either all illegal, or none of them are. Many forensic scientists may wish to use a uniform prior distribution, sometimes

---

[†] European Network of Forensic Institutes
[‡] Pronounced gamma.

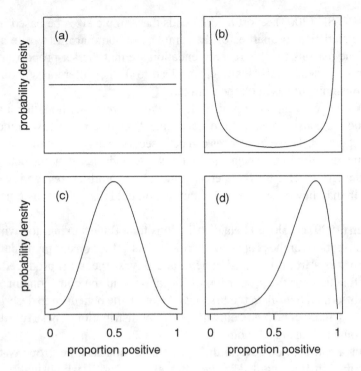

Figure 16.3 Four different beta distributions which could represent a prior belief about the proportions of positive units in a consignment. (a) has both $\alpha = 1$ and $\beta = 1$ which gives a uniform distribution. (b) has $\alpha = 0.5$ and $\beta = 0.5$. It takes the form of a U which could be used to indicate that the prior belief that the consignment is most likely to have no illicit units, or, the entire consignment will be illegal. (c) has $\alpha = 4$ and $\beta = 4$ which indicates that there is a reasonably strong prior belief for the proportion of illegal units is 0.50. (d) has $\alpha = 6$ and $\beta = 2$ which would suggest a fairly strong prior belief that the proportion of illicit units is 0.75. Vertical scales have been omitted for clarity, the vertical scales for the prior density functions and the posterior density functions are *not* necessarily equal

known as an *ignorance prior*, which means that the true proportion of illegal units is as likely to be at any particular proportion as any other. This occurs when $\alpha = 1$ and $\beta = 1$ and the prior is a straight line as with Figure 16.3(A).

The process of estimating the proportion of positive units in a consignment of suspected illegal drugs shares many similarities with coin tossing. Let us say that from observation of 5 units from a consignment of 90 units, four contain illicit substances (m), and one (n) does not. The beta posterior density function for the proportion of positives, θ, in the consignment is given by:

$$f(\theta \mid \alpha + m, \beta + n) = \frac{\theta^{m+\alpha-1}(1-\theta)^{n-\beta-1}}{\mathbf{B}(m+\alpha, n+\beta)} \tag{38}$$

This is calculated in Figure 16.4 for the prior distributions depicted in Figure 16.3.

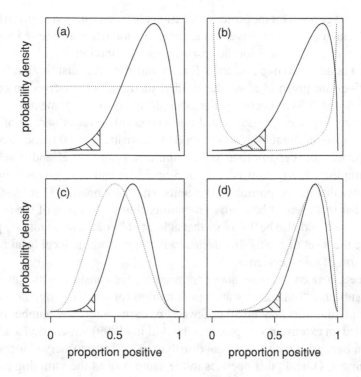

Figure 16.4 Posterior distributions (solid lines) for the observation that out of a sample of five units in a consignment, four contain narcotic substances the lower 5% tail of the posterior distribution is hatched. The prior probabilities (dotted lines in this figure) are from Figure 16.3. (a) with prior parameters $\alpha = 1$ $\beta = 1$ after the information of four positives and one negative we can say that there is a 95% probability that 41% or more of the consignment contains narcotics. (b) for prior parameters $\alpha = 0.5$ $\beta = 0.5$ the posterior distribution tells us that there is a 95% probability that 43% of the consignment is illicit. For (c) with prior parameters $\alpha = 4$ $\beta = 4$ the posterior tells us there is a 95% probability that 39% or more of the consignment is illegal, and (d) with prior parameters $\alpha = 6$ $\beta = 2$ the posterior tells us that there is a 95% probability that at least 56% of the consignment contains narcotics. Vertical scales have been omitted for clarity, the vertical scales for the prior density functions and the posterior density functions are not necessarily equal

The beta posterior distribution can be treated in the same manner as any other probability density function in that areas corresponding to ordinates can be calculated, or more specifically ordinates corresponding to areas, to calculate a lower bound for the proportion of units containing the substance in question given the sample. For example, if a uniform prior is adopted in the example above then the posterior distribution is the solid line in Figure 16.4A, and there would be a 95% probability that 41% or more of the consignment would contain the illicit substance.

Computation of the above probability density functions requires a computer. However, it is relatively simple, given suitable computer software, to calculate tables of any percentage point for the posterior function given in Equation 38 given the number of units which assayed positive for the drug, the number which tested negative, and the parameters of α and β for the desired prior distribution.

Such a table is given in Appendix E for a uniform prior distribution. The number of positives are given in rows, the number of negatives observed in columns for 90%, 95% and 99% respectively. For example, a large consignment comprising 100 sub-units of suspected drugs is seized, and a randomly selected sample of 5 sub-units assayed. If five of the sub-units are found to be positive, and 0 found to be negative, and it thought most appropriate to use a uniform prior ($\alpha = 1$ and $\beta = 1$), then by consulting the table in Appendix E for 5 positives and 0 negatives there is a 90% probability that the proportion of sub-units which are positive is at least 0.68. This means that there would be a 90% probability that 68 or more of the sub-units are positive. We could also be 99% sure that at least 46% of the sub-units are positive. In this case the level of probability desired will depend on the local legal requirement for this sort of assay evidence.

The beta-beta calculations above are accurate for consignments with large numbers of sub-units, but are only an approximation for small consignments where the number of sub-units may be 50 or fewer. For cases where the number of sub-units are limited an extension was proposed by Aitkin (1999) which used a mixed distribution, a beta prior with a binomial distribution for the unobserved members of the consignment. Overall, this operates in the same way as the sampling above, but is specifically tailored to give accurate results for small consignments.

A further extension is to the quantity of illegal substance in a consignment. This problem is addressed in Aitken and Lucy (2002), and uses another formulation of the beta method described above. In this measurements are taken of the weight of several items of the suspicious consignment, and take the mean and standard deviation of those measurements. A beta prior for the proportion of the consignment thought to be illegal is then combined with a t-density representing the uncertainty in weight, and beta representing uncertainty in the number of positives, to produce a posterior density function for the weight of the substance in the remaining units.

16.4 Concluding comments

Sample size estimation can sometimes be difficult, not because it is particularly problematic mathematically, but because there must be some clear idea of what is to be established from the sample, and some notion of the likely results from the observations. It is not possible to calculate sample sizes without knowing anything about the distributions of measurements underlying the samples.

The question of random sampling has not really arisen above, but it is nonetheless an important one. Quite often in practical science choice of sample is not really something which arises: the scientist just has to make do with what they are given, or can take, without regard to the finer points of sampling theory. In these cases it is worthwhile considering whether the sample has been collected with some obvious biasing factor. For instance, the specimens making up the sample are those which caught the eye of the individual gathering the sample, it could well be that the sample is biased in some way, that is, the sample could comprise, larger, smaller, or specimens of a different colour or appearance to the rest. Even if the sample varies in some systematic way to the population this may not be of importance as it is systematic variation in the property of interest which is of importance.

The ideal random sample would consist of each item in the population being labelled, then a random number generated which would select each member of the population with uniform probability. This is simple for small to moderate size populations, but becomes impractical in consignments of 20 000 sub-units, and it must be left to the ingenuity of the forensic scientist to think of ways to approach as close as possible to a true random sample. Practical guidance to sampling can be found in Barnett (1974), a more complete reference being available from Cochran (1977).

Review questions

1. In an extensive study of infant organ weights Thompson and Cohle (2004, Table 1) give the mean brain weight for 9-month-old infants which are said to have been the victim of sudden infant death syndrome (SIDS) as 953g with a standard deviation of 240g. They based this on a sample of five infants. What would the sample size have to be able to be 99% confident that the mean is $953 \pm 100\,g$?

2. Thompson and Cohle (2004, Table 1) also report that for non-SIDS infant deaths the mean brain weights are 905 g with a standard deviation of 238 g. This is based on a sample of seven infants. If the differences between the SIDS sample and non-SIDS infants mean brain weights are reflected in the wider populations what would be a reasonable sample size to detect that difference with a two-sample t-test?

3. A seizure of 348 packets of suspected cocaine have been taken from the bag of a suspect. The drugs examiner has tested ten for cocaine and found it present in nine of the packages. How many packages are you 99% sure are positive for cocaine from the bag?

17

Epilogue

Statistical science has been undergoing a fundamental change since the early 1990s from frequentist implementations and interpretations, to more and more Bayesian approaches. This change has been enabled by statisticians' increased ability to make complex calculations in highly multivariate spaces, and driven by data and propositions of greater complexity. It should not be thought that classical type hypothesis tests are in some sense wrong. They are not. They have exactly the same firm grounding in probability theory that later approaches have. It all depends on where and how the classical tests are applied, and the interpretation one expects to be able to place upon their results. Hypothesis type testing of data is perfectly appropriate in the laboratory where there may not be a long run of sufficiently similar events to justify a frequentist interpretation, but for which such a long run is certainly possible as more experiments can always be performed. However, evidence in law has little provision for classes of events; each case must be decided upon the singular nature of its evidence. There is no long run of events possible in law, so unless the whole notion that evidence has a measurable value is to be discarded, interpretations of evidence which require that probability is based upon long runs has to be replaced with some other idea. The only other plausible contender is that probability is a statement of belief.

It is a combination of this, and the fact that, historically, evidence evaluation techniques have been developed at a time when more Bayesian methods were also being developed, which explains the dichotomous structure of this book. Classical testing approaches have been treated here as suitable for the laboratory, and have been in common use since the early years of the twentieth century. Bayesian techniques tend to be used for evidential evaluation, and have become more common in the latter years of the 20th century. This is not by any means a true dichotomy. Bayesian methods are available to the laboratory scientist (Lee, 2004) and may replace common hypothesis tests in the next few decades due to ease of interpretation, greater

Introduction to Statistics for Forensic Scientists David Lucy
© 2005 John Wiley & Sons, Ltd.

flexibility when applied to complex data, and the fact that Bayesian approaches constitute the greater part of the development of statistical science at the moment.

The development of statistics applied to forensic science mirrors developments seen in the wider world of statistical science. A greater emphasis on Bayesian methods, non-parametric distributions, and the analysis of complex multi-multifaceted data are all features of current ideas from the statistical community. The remainder of this chapter will outline three of the more prominent of these developments.

17.1 Graphical models and Bayesian Networks

Graphical models and Bayesian networks are two interconnected themes in statistical science. A graphical model at its simplest is a way of representing dependencies between multivariate data. Bayesian networks have graphical models as a fundamental component, but feature additional rules and methods which allow a full representation of complex data, interdependencies between variables in those data, and ways of calculating probabilities for outcomes of interest from those complex data.

Graphical models

A simple graphical model can be illustrated from the morphine redistribution data given by Gerostamoulos and Drummer (2000). In Table 6.7 we calculated the partial correlations between M3 measured on admission (denoted A), M3 measured during post-mortem examination (denoted B), and free morphine measured during postmortem examination (denoted C). The upper triangle of the partial correlation table is reproduced below.

	M3 admission (A)	M3 post mortem (B)	Free morphine (C)
M3 admission (A)	1.000	0.811	0.113
M3 post mortem(B)	–	1.000	0.011
Free morphine (C)	–	–	1.000

A graphical model of all dependencies for variables A, B, and C is given in Figure17.1(a). The circled letters represent the variables, and are termed *nodes*. The arrows between the variables are called *edges* and represent the dependency between the two variables. For instance, there is an arrow between nodes A and B, which represents the correlation of 0.811 between M3 on admission and M3 at post-mortem examination. The direction of the arrow in this case suggests that M3 at post-mortem examination *depends on* M3 on admission. The choice of edge direction in this case comes from background knowledge of morphine redistribution, but in

(a)

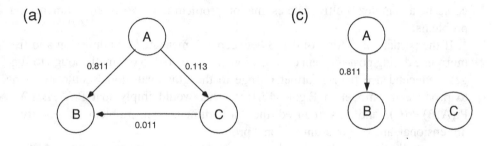

(c)

(b)

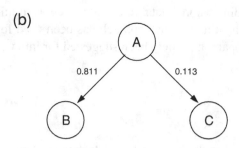

Figure 17.1 Some graphical models representing possible dependence structures from the partial correlation matrix for Gerostamoulos and Drummer's (2000) morphine redistribution data. (a) is the full model taking into account all dependencies between M3 on admission, M3 at post-mortem examination and free morphine measured during post-mortem examination. (b) is where the correlation between M3 measured during post-mortem examination is considered independent of free morphine, and (c) is where M3 measured on admission is considered independent of free morphine observed during post-mortem examination

more ambiguous cases, where there is a larger graphical model with more nodes, there are rules which define the placement and direction of edges to make the model satisfy criteria of directed and acyclic (Whittaker, 1990).

If one wished to calculate the probability for a particular value of these three variables then it would be necessary to calculate $\Pr(A, B, C)$. Usually for three variables this would not be a problem, however, were too few data available then one might wish to think about the problem of calculating a probability from a three-dimensional space as a product of multiple independent lower dimensional probabilities.

This could be achieved by examining Figure 17.1(a) and noting that the correlation between free morphine during post-mortem examination has a very low partial correlation with M3 at post-mortem examination. This partial correlation could be considered low enough for free morphine during post-mortem examinations, and M3 at post-mortem examinations (variables A and B) to be thought of as independent. A graphical model of this dependence structure would be represented as Figure 17.1(b), and would imply that $\Pr(A, B, C) = \Pr(A|B)\Pr(A|C)$. Here we have broken what could be a complex multivariate estimation problem into two smaller dimensional problems.

If the partial correlation of 0.113 between M3 measured on admission and free morphine during post-mortem examination is considered to be small enough to suggest independence then a further change to the graphical model could be made to produce the model in Figure 17.1(c). This would imply that $\Pr(A, B, C) = \Pr(A|B)\Pr(C)$, and has reduced the three-dimensional problem to one two-dimensional, and one one-dimensional problems.

Essentially here graphical models have been used to reduce the number of dependencies within a complex dataset. This allows probabilities which would have had to have been calculated from high dimensional data, to be calculated as multiple independent lower dimensional probabilities. This approach has been used for biological estimation (Lucy *et al.*, 2002), and has lately been suggested for into use in forensic science (Aitken *et al.*, 2005).

Bayesian networks

A Bayesian network is similar in structure to the graphical models described above with edges representing dependencies, however the composition of the nodes is different. In a Bayesian network each node will typically represent a *real world* state, and will comprise a set of mutually exclusive, and exhaustive, state values. The value ascribed to each state value will be a probability, the probabilities for each node sum to one. For illustration a typical node might consist of the state values 'guilty' and 'innocent', each state value might then have a probability associated with it. Another node might consist of the world state 'hard evidence', which might have the states 'yes' and 'no'. A link indicating some sort of causal dependency between the two could then be formed which represents a way in which changes in the 'hard evidence' node affect the 'guilty/innocent' node. When the network is run, changes in one node will be propagated through all nodes in the network, typically there will be one node of greatest interest; in the example above it may be the 'guilty/innocent' node, which will constitute the output of the network.

A Bayesian network, as illustrated above, with just two nodes is simple instantiation of Bayes' theorem. Where Bayes' networks come into their own is where the structure of the propositions is more complicated. Examples can be seen in Fenton and Neil (2000) where errors of reasoning were investigated with a Bayesian network, and Dawid *et al.* (2000) for more general applications to forensic science. However, a further advantage is that Bayesian networks can be constructed for single pieces of evidence; these networks can be easily combined together to produce a larger network (Aitken *et al.*, 2003) which combines evidence from different evidence types from a case to allow all information to be considered in a natural, but mathematically rigorous way.

17.2 Kernel density estimation

A kernel density function is simply another way of estimating a probability density function from observed data. Statisticians have always been aware that not all data can be modelled using simple parametric distributions, but until it became easy to do the calculations with a computer it was very difficult to use anything else.

Kernel density approaches exist for discrete and continuous data types and can most easily be described as a *sum of bumps* (Silverman, 1986). Figure 17.2 is a kernel density estimate of the array $x = \{2, 4, 5\}$. Each of the values has a small component distribution associated with it. In this case the distributions are normal in form, are centred around 2, 4 and 5 respectively, and have a standard deviation $h = 0.5$. These are shown in Figure 17.2 as a dashed line, the centres being shown as vertical dotted lines. The individual component distributions are simply summed to produce an estimate of the sample density function. This is shown as the solid line in Figure 17.2.

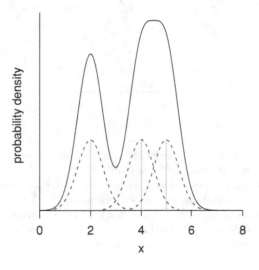

Figure 17.2   A sum of bumps illustration of a kernel density estimate of the array $x = \{2, 4, 5\}$. Each point is represented by a small density function; in this case the component density functions are normal in form, and are shown as the dashed lines about their central (dotted line) values. The sample density function is then made by summing the densities for all the points resulting in the density function marked as the solid line. The component density functions, and the kernel density estimate are on different vertical scales.

The parameter h is called a window width, and affects the smoothness of the final density estimate. A small value of h leads to a 'spiky' estimate, whereas a large value of h gives a very smooth density estimate. The theory behind selecting a suitable window width is extensive, but various strategies can be employed such as each value having its own value of h, and allowing h to vary continuously throughout the range of x (Wand and Jones, 1995).

The effect of varying the window width (h) can be seen in Figure 17.3. This is for the Δ^9-THC data given in Figure 4.2. Three values have been used for h. For the density function represented by the dashed line, h has been set to 0.2%, for the dotted line, $h = 1.0$%. The density function where $h = 1.0$% is considerably smoother than that where $h = 0.2$%, and approximates the modelled normal density from Figure 4.2. The distribution represented by the solid line is calculated using $h = 0.5$% which theory suggests is an optimal value for these data, and lies between the two extremes of 'spikeyness' and smoothness respectively given by the other estimates.

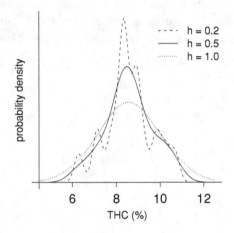

Figure 17.3   Three kernel density estimates of the distribution of Δ^9-THC (%) in marijuana seizures from 1986 from the simulated data from Table 2.2. The distribution represented by the dashed line was calculated using a window width (h) of 0.2%, that represented by the dotted line h was set to 1.0%. The dashed line represents a less smooth distribution than that represented by the dotted line, and is undersmoothed. The dotted line is a little oversmoothed. The distribution represented by the solid line is calculated using $h = 0.5$% which is an optimum value suggested by theory for the window width for these particular data

Kernel density estimates of distributions can be calculated for multiple dimensions, and where multivariate data have interdepedencies, and are being seen as a way of calculating probabilities without making many distributional assumptions where some other distribution, such as the normal, cannot be shown to describe the data adequately.

17.3 Multivariate continuous matching

Quite often, dependent on what sort of object is being examined, the observations on objects from forensic objects are multivariate and continuous. An ideal exemplar would be the chemical composition of some material such as glass. If a window has been broken during the commission of a crime, and a suspect is apprehended, and found to have some glass fragments on their clothing, what is the value of evidence for the measurements of elemental composition used to compare the fragments of glass from the suspect to those of the window?

Many previous attempts have used simply the difference between each measurement measured on some form of modified two sample t-test. For example, Koons and Buscaglia (2002) examined a number of variables and used a test based upon a t-distribution between multiple measurements from the same fragment. If any measurement was excluded at some level of significance, then the two glass fragments were declared not to be a match. The problem with this approach, as with all hypothesis testing approaches as discussed in Section 8.4, is that it is undoubtedly capable of excluding fragments which do not match, but it is far from telling you what a match means.

In fact with data on a continuous scale, the notion of *match* is entirely artificial, being created with arbitrary boundaries. If the underlying variable is continuous then no two pieces can have exactly the same composition. They can be close, but not exactly the same in the same way that a red ball is categorically similar to another red ball. In other words, we only have varying degrees of similarity and dissimilarity.

A solution to this problem can be thought about by considering how a piece of glass found at a crimescene (α) is compared by measuring Sn and Fe concentrations to a fragment of glass found in the possession of a suspect (β). Due to within fragment variability and measurement variability, the two measurements are unlikely to be exactly the same. In fact with multiple measurements a distribution can be built up for the similarity between the two pieces of glass in relation to the distributions for their respective measurements. However, this is not the entire story. It tells us nothing about how many other pieces of glass could fit the description. Figure 17.4 gives a graphical illustration of this where two points are placed against a background population of measurements from similar items. Figure 17.4(a) shows the two points as quite similar, however, the value of the distance represented by the arrow has to be conditioned on how many other possible matches there could be, so the evidence that these two points represent the same item is lower than the position were the two arranged as in (B). Figure 17.4(b) shows where there are fewer points in the local background, hence the value of the observation of proximity to each other is higher than in Figure 17.4(a) for the hypothesis that the observations were made on on objects coming from the same proximal source. The same is true in Figure 17.4(c) and Figure 17.4(d), which have a larger distance between the two objects represented in the space, but maintain the same positions relative to the background population.

This sort of approach was first suggested by Lindley (1977) for univariate continuous data. Its application to the analysis of multivariate data is outlined by Curran *et al.* (2000) and more latterly by Aitken and Lucy (2004). So far results have been encouraging in that in experiments on a dataset of glass elemental compositions the likelihood ratio based methods record fewer *false positives* than any other type of technique used to compare this data type. Unfortunately the data requirements are

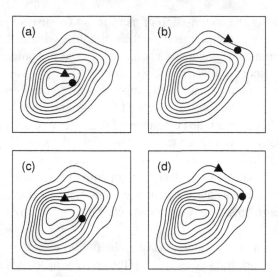

Figure 17.4 Four possible pairs of points relative to a wider population in a two-dimensional space. Points with observations in the two-dimensional space can be represented by the solid circle and the solid triangle; the background density is represented by the contours. In (a) the circle and triangle are close together, however, the background density is high. This means that many possible pairs of observations will have the same proximity to each other, so the evidential value that these observations are selected from the same object is low. This contrasts with (b) where the distance between the observations represented by the circle and triangle is small, and they are at a point relative to the background distribution where there are few possible pairs of points. This means that the evidential value for identity between the two objects will be high. In (e) the observations represented by the circle and triangle are more widely spaced than in (a), and the background density is high, so the evidential value for the two points coming from the same item is lower than for the position in (a). In (d) the two points are even more widely spaced than in (b), so the evidential value for identity between the items represented by the circle and triangle will be lower than for (b). However, there are few points in the background distribution. It is possible to say that the position in (a) has a higher evidential value for identity of the two objects than that in (c), and (b) than (d). But without performing the calculations it is not possible to compare the position seen in (b) with (c), or (c) and (d)

much higher than simply looking at the proximity between points, and the calculations are far harder. The computational aspects can be addressed by software, but the amount of background data needed, and the consideration of what constitutes a suitable background population, will place extra burdens on forensic scientists. There is, however, little choice than to adopt these types of methods as to rely on purely proximity based measures of evidential value would be to commit the methodological error termed the *different level* error (See 13.2) where proximity alone is confused with identity.

Appendix A
Worked solutions to questions

Solutions to Chapter 2

1. A DNA profile has discrete stages which relate to the alleles of the specific type at the locus, so it could be ordinal, but alleles tend just to be used as a classification, so therefore we could also say it is categorical.

2. The five measurements from each fragment are a sample of a nearly infinite population of measurements I could take of refractive index from each fragment. The 20 fragments are a sample of a finite population of possible fragments from the pane of glass.

3. Indeed it is.

4. It should not be as all adults include men and women, men have a greater mean height than women, so the distribution should be bimodal.

5. The variable sex is being used as a factor.

6. First we are given the information $X = \{16, 17, 21, 21, 21, 23, 23\}$.

    (a) Evaluate just means 'find the value of'. In this case it is $x_1 + x_3$. Looking above $x_1 = 16$ and $x_3 = 21$, so $16 + 21 = 37$.

    (b) $\sum_1^3 x = x_1 + x_2 + x_3 = 16 + 17 + 21 = 54$

    (c) $\bar{x}$ is the mean of x. This is $\sum_1^7 x = 16 + 17 + 21 + 21 + 21 + 23 + 23 = 142$ divided by $n = 7$, which is $142/7 = 20.28$.

    (d) The median is the middle value of the ordered series of x. As x has seven elements then the median is the fourth element of the ordered series, which is 21.

(e) The mode is the most frequently occurring value in x, which is 21.

(f) The variance is nearly the mean of the squares of the distances of the elements of x from the mean of x, that is:

$$\text{var}(x) = \frac{\sum_{i=1}^{7}(x_i - \bar{x})^2}{n - 1}$$

$\bar{x} = 20.28$ so $x - \bar{x} = \{-4.29, -3.29, 0.71, 0.71, 0.71, 2.71, 2.71\}$,   which squared is $\{18.37, 10.80, 0.51, 0.51, 0.51, 7.37, 7.37\}$, summing $\sum_{i=1}^{7}(x_i - \bar{x})^2 = 45.44$, and dividing by $n - 1 = 6$ is 7.57.

Solutions to Chapter 3

1. In the National Lottery balls numbered $1, 2, \ldots, 49$ are sampled. In order to win the jackpot you must have guessed correctly all six balls drawn, the order in which they are drawn is unimportant. The National Lottery makes sure that all balls are equally likely to be drawn, and that non-replacement independence is maintained between successive balls. For the first ball I have to guess correctly one ball from 49, so the probability is $1/49$ of getting the first ball right. For the second ball I still have to guess one ball correctly, but this time, because the first ball is not replaced I have only 48 balls to choose from. The third ball I have to choose one from 47 and so on until all the balls have been selected.

   However, ordering is not important, so in the first selection I can choose any of the six which will be selected from the 49 available. For the second I can select any of the five remaining from the now 48 available, and so on. So I can choose a winning selection with probability $p = 6/49 \times 5/48 \times 4/47 \times 3/46 \times 2/45 \times 1/44 \approx 7.151 \times 10^{-8}$ from a single ticket. With my five tickets I have five opportunities to get the combination right, thus I have a $5 \times 7, 151 \times 10^{-8}$ which is ≈ 1 in 2.8 million chance of winning.

2. The probability of *not* winning the lottery is $1-$ the probability of winning. The probability of winning is above, and the probability of not winning is close to 1 ($p = 0.9999996$).

3. In the dice game you can either win or not win. If it can be assumed that the dice is fair, and six sided, this can be considered using a binomial model which is:

$$Pr(X = x) = \frac{n!}{x!(n - x)!} \, p^x (1 - p)^{(n-x)}$$

   The dice are numbered $1, 2, \ldots, 6$, so the probability of throwing one six is $1/6$. x in this case is the requirement to get three sixes from $n = 5$ throws. Substituting into the above:

$$Pr(X = 3) = \frac{5!}{3!(5 - 3)!} \, (1/6)^3 (1 - (1/6))^{(5-3)}$$

$$= \frac{120}{6(2)!} \, (1/6)^3 (5/6)^{(2)}$$

$$= \frac{120}{12} \, (1/216)(25/36)$$

$$= 0.032.$$

which gives you a 3.2% chance of winning, which is very much better then the National Lottery, but still is not good.

4. If the THC content of marijuana seized in 1986 is to be $\leq 8\%$ then it is the sum of the probabilities for it being 6% to 8%, so from Table 3.3 this is $6.0 \rightarrow 6.5$ which is 0.05 plus $6.5 \rightarrow 7.0$ being 0.00 plus $7.0 \rightarrow 7.5$ is 0.10 and $7.5 \rightarrow 8.0$ which is 0.10, summing $0.05 + 0.00 + 0.01 + 0.01 = 0.25$, or 25%.

Solutions to Chapter 4

1. The ten marijuana consignments have mean 9.5%, and variance 8.9.

   (a) As the variance is 8.9 and the standard deviation is the square root of the variance, this means $sd = 2.98\%$. The difference between 10% and 9.5% is 0.5%, which is $0.50/2.98 = 0.17$ standard deviations. From Appendix B 0.17 standard deviations have 0.5675 of the area underneath it. 15% is 5.5% from the sample mean, which is $5.5/2.98 = 1.85$ standard deviations. From Appendix B 1.85 standard deviations have 0.9678 of the area underneath it. So to find the area between 1.85 and 0.17 standard deviations we simply take 0.5675 from $0.9678 = 0.4003$. In other words the probability that the THC content is between 10% and 15% is 40%.
   (b) The standard error of the mean is $2.98\% / \sqrt{10} = 0.942\%$.
   (c) For a 99% confidence interval we need 1% of the area in Appendix B to be in both tails, this means that each tail should have 0.5%. Therefore the area required in Appendix B is 0.9950 which by inspection of Appendix B corresponds to 2.58 standard deviations. So the interval is given by $9.5\% \pm 2.58 \times 2.98\%$ which is $9.5\% \pm 7.69\% = 1.81\% \rightarrow 17.19\%$.

2. The heroin consignments have mean 19.38%, and variance 10.95%.

   (a) As the variance is 10.95% the standard deviation is 3.31%, so the standard error of the mean is $3.31\%/\sqrt{10} = 1.05\%$. The distribution for the mean is $19.38\% \pm t \times 1.046$, as there are ten observations in the sample the degrees of freedom $= 9$. Looking at the 95% column in Appendix C the corresponding value of t is 2.262. So the 95% confidence interval for the mean is $19.38\% \pm 2.262 \times 1.05\%$ which is $19.38\% \pm 2.37\% = 17.00\% \rightarrow 21.76\%$
   (b) Very similar to above, but this time use the 99% column in Appendix C to get a value of $t = 3.250$. Thus, the interval is $19.38\% \pm 3.250 \times 1.05\%$, giving a 99% confidence interval from 15.97% to 22.97%.

3. The mean of the widths of the sample of the dog hairs found in association with the victim was $\bar{x}_1 = 49.71 \, \mu m$, with variance $54.08 \, \mu m^2$. The sample from the suspect's

dog $\bar{x}_2 = 37.86\,\mu$m, with variance $54.76\,\mu$m^3. As the two variances are similar then homogeneity of variances is assumed.

We wish to examine whether $\bar{x} - \bar{y} = 11.84\,\mu$m represents a real difference at some predefined level of significance. We know the distribution of the difference of the two means is (Equation 8 on p. 37):

$$se(\bar{x}_1 - \bar{x}_2) = \hat{s}\sqrt{\frac{1}{n_1} + \frac{1}{n_2}}$$

where:

$$\hat{s} = \sqrt{\frac{(n_1 - 1)s_1^2 + (n_2 - 1)s_2^2}{n_1 + n_2 - 2}}$$

$s_1^2 = 54.08$ and $s_2^2 = 54.76$, $n_1 = n_2 = 5$, so substituting into the above equation to calculate an estimate of the pooled variance $\hat{s} = 7.38$. Calculating $se(\bar{x}_1 - \bar{x}_2)$ from above we have a pooled estimate of the standard error for $(\bar{x}_1 - \bar{x}_2)$ of $0.6324 \times 7.38 = 4.67$.

For $n_1 + n_2 - 2 = 8$ degrees of freedom t is at 2.306 standard errors at 95% confidence, so the 95% confidence interval for the difference in the two means is $11.84 \pm 2.306 \times 4.67 = 11.84 \pm 10.76$, giving a 95% confidence interval of $1.08 \rightarrow 22.60$. This interval does not include zero, so at 95% confidence one would exclude the suspect's dog as being the origin of the hairs on the victim acquired during the commission of the crime.

Examining the difference at 99% confidence for 8 degrees of freedom we find a suitable value of t of 3.355, so at 99% confidence the interval is $11.84 \pm 3.355 \times 4.67 = 11.84 \pm 15.66$, giving a confidence interval of $-3.82 \rightarrow 27.50$. This interval does include zero so would not exclude the hairs found on the victim's clothing as coming from the suspect's dog.

The seeming contradiction between saying that the hairs came from different sources at 95% confidence, and saying they came from the same source at 99% confidence is one of the difficulties inherent in using significance type tests to evaluate forensic evidence. The contradiction can be resolved by considering the meaning of significance in this context. The probability to which 95% and 99% confidence refer is related to 5% and 1% significance, and is the probability of falsely rejecting the *null hypothesis* when it is in fact true. The *null hypothesis* in this case is that the two samples of dog hair widths are drawn from the same population of dog hair widths. Now the probability makes more sense as the null hypothesis is rejected, and we reject the null hypoth that the widths came from the same population more easily when we are willing falsely to reject the hypothesis that they are the same with greater probability. It should be noted that a t-test as performed here tells us nothing about the probabilities of the hairs coming from the same dog.

The answer to the question is that it is possible the hairs came from the same dog, and, to exclude the suspect's dog on the basis of these samples, we would be making a mistake between 1% and 5% of the time.

4. If we can assume that each donor on each occasion form independent observations this can be treated as a paired experiment. If so a one-sample t-test is an appropriate

means to examine the differences between in cell extraction between water and PBS.

Cells water (x_1)	Cells PBS (x_1)	Difference (d)	$d - \bar{d}$	$(d - \bar{d})^2$
1215	1284	−39	177.78	31604.94
1319	1063	256	472.78	223518.83
568	1138	−570	−352.22	124765.94
1675	1666	9	225.778	50975.60
1912	3209	−1297	−1080.22	1166880.05
1982	2986	−1004	−787.22	619718.83
3103	3209	−106	110.78	12271.72
1969	1325	344	560.78	314471.72
3135	2679	456	672.78	452629.94
$\bar{x}_1 = 1845.33$	$\bar{x}_2 = 2062.11$	$\bar{d} = -216.78$		$\sum = 2996838$

The table gives the means of the observations, the mean of the differences, and the sum of squared deviations for a sample of nine paired observations. The mean of differences is −216.78, the PBS seeming to extract marginally more than just water. The sum of squared deviations is 2996838 so the variance is $2996838/(n-1) = 2996838/8 = 374604.7$, so the standard deviation is $\sqrt{374604.7} = 612.05$. The standard error of the mean is therefore $612.05/\sqrt{9} = 612.05/3 = 204.02$.

We find that 2.306 is a suitable value of t by looking up in Appendix C t at 95% confidence for $9 - 1 = 8$ degrees of freedom. Therefore a 95% confidence interval for the differences in means is $-216.78 \pm (2.306 \times 204.02) = -216.78 \pm 470.46$, so the 95% confidence interval is $-687.24 \rightarrow 253.68$.

This confidence interval includes zero as a possible valve for the mean of the differences, and thus there is insufficent evidence of a real difference between the numbers of cells extracted in water, and numbers extracted in PBS.

Solutions to Chapter 5

1. For convenience McNamara and Morton's (2004) Table 2 is reproduced here:

Year	Murders
1987	437
1988	468
1989	480
1990	545
1991	584
1992	563
1993	539
1994	570
1995	501
1996	496

The question was: is there any evidence to support the notion that the number of murders are related to year?

A single sample χ^2 test is appropriate here. In Chapter 5 we did not explicitly cover the single sample variant of the χ^2 test, but after the two-sample test it is trivially easy.

The first thing to do is to think about some idea for generating the number of murders which may be expected per year. In the absence of any further information the best expected measure of the number of murders is the mean of the number of murders in the sample period, which is 518.3 murders. We then substitute the data values and expected score into Equation 10 on p. 46 to gain the following table where O means observed and E is expected:

Murders	$O - E$	$(O - E)^2$	$(O - E)^2/E$
437	−81.3	6609.69	12.75
468	−50.3	2530.09	4.88
480	−38.3	1466.89	2.83
545	26.7	712.89	1.38
584	65.7	4316.49	8.33
563	44.7	1998.09	3.86
539	20.7	428.49	0.83
570	51.7	2672.89	5.16
501	−17.3	299.29	0.58
496	−22.3	497.29	0.96
mean = 518.3			$\sum$ 41.54

So the value for χ^2 is 41.54. This is compared with the value for χ^2 for $n - 1$ degrees of freedom in the table in Appendix D. n in this case is simply the number of categories, which is 10, so $10 - 1 = 9$. A value for χ^2 with 9 degrees of freedom at 99% level of confidence is 21.67. The calculated value of χ^2 is 41.54 which is considerably larger than the tabulated χ^2 at 99% confidence, meaning that the calculated value of χ^2 is some distance into one of the extreme tails of the distribution.

This provides some evidence that the murder rate in Virginia is related in some way to the year, or, to put it more simply, that the murder rate in Virginia between 1987 and 1996 could not be considered uniform.

McNamara and Morton (2004) compared the murder rate for non-sexually motivated murder with that for serial sexual related murder for the time period and found an unusually low frequency for serial sexual related murder in Virginia.

2. Pittella and Gusmao (2003, Table 2) of DVI and DAI injuries is:

	DAI	
DVI	present	absent
present	14	0
absent	82	24

The first thing we may wish to know is: is there a significant association between presence and absence of DVI, and presence and absence of DAI? A χ^2 measure of association may be appropriate. Calculating from the row and column totals the expected values the following table is obtained (expected values in parentheses):

| | DAI | | |
DVI	present	absent	total
present	14(11.2)	0(2.8)	14
absent	82(84.8)	24(21.2)	106
total	96	24	120

The value of zero in the upper right-hand cell in the table may give cause for concern, however each expected value is greater than 1, and the mean of the expected values is 30, which is larger than the value of 5 which would put the use of the χ^2 test in danger.

From Equation 10 on p. 46 we have a value of $\chi^2 = 3.96$. The table has two rows and two columns, this 1 degree of freedom [(rows $-$ 1) $\times$ (columns -1)]. From the table in Appendix D the ordinate for χ^2 with 1 degree of freedom is 3.84 at 95% confidence and 6.64 at 99% confidence. The calculated value of $\chi^2 = 3.96$ is marginally significant at the 5% level, but not at all at the 1% level.

As this is a 2×2 table, and we wish to know about the nature of the relationship between DVI and DAI, then Yule's Q might seem a suitable additional measure to the χ^2 test.

From Equation 11 on p. 49:

$$Q = \frac{AD - BC}{AD + BC}$$

which from the table $A = 12$, $B = 0$, $C = 82$, and $D = 24$. So:

$$Q = \frac{AD - BC}{AD + BC} = \frac{(12 \times 24) - (0 \times 82)}{(12 \times 24) + (0 \times 82)} = \frac{288}{288} = 1$$

The problem here is that we have a 'complete' association between the presence and absence of DAI when DVI is presence. That is, DAI is never absent when DVI is present. This makes our value of Yules $Q = 1$.

Due to their relationship Pittella and Gusmao (2003) suggested both forms of brain lesion have in part a common mechanism for their formation, and that possibly they should be seen as part of a continuity of brain lesion, rather than as separate entities.

3. De Kinder's (2002) firearm data are reproduced with row and column totals in the table.

Firearm	Project	Casework	Total
0.177 air	3	12	15
0.22	68	23	91
6.35 Browning	8	14	22
7.65 Browning	11	41	52
9 mm parabellum	17	32	49
total	107	122	229

One way in which we can think about whether the types of firearms seen in the project, and those seen in casework are significantly different is by examining the evidence for an association between gun type, and project and casework.

The expected values for each cell can be calculated by the product of the corresponding rows and columns divided by the total for all rows and columns. For the top left-hand cell the row total is therefore 15, the column total is 107, and the grand total is 229, so the expected value is $(15 \times 107)/229 = 7.00$. The scores and expected values are given in the table. The expected values are in parentheses.

3 (7.00)	12 (7.99)
68 (42.52)	23 (48.48)
8 (10.28)	14 (11.72)
11 (24.30)	41 (27.70)
17 (22.89)	32 (26.10)

Substituting these values into Equation 10 on p. 46 the value for χ^2 is 50.4. There are 4 [(rows − 1) × (columns −1)] degrees of freedom. Examination of the table in Appendix D gives a value of 9.488 at 95% confidence, and 13.277 at 99% confidence. Our calculated value of ≈ 50 is more extreme than either of these, meaning that there are significant differences at a level less than 31% between the two samples.

De Kinder (2002) outlined work on a test project on all seized firearms from an area of Belgium to evaluate the efficacy of a ballistic database. De Kinder pointed to the discrepancies between firearms available to the authorities for examination, and those actually used for criminal offences.

4. Gülekon and Turgut's (2003) data are reproduced here.

Type	Women	Men	Total
type I	427	89	516
type II	52	94	146
type III	21	317	338
total	500	500	1000

The expected frequencies for each cell can be calculated by multiplying the corresponding row and column totals divided by the grand total, so the expected frequency for the top left-hand cell is $(516 \times 500)/1000$.

Type	Women	Men
type I	427 (258)	89 (258)
type II	52 (73)	94 (73)
type III	21 (169)	317 (169)

Substituting values from the table into Equation 10 on p. 46 the value for χ^2 is 492.7. With 2 columns and 3 rows there are 2 df. The table in Appendix E gives a value fo x^2 5.991 at 95% confidence, and 9.210 at 99% confidence. Our calculated value of ≈ 490 is more extreme than either of tabulated values, meaning that there is a significant association at a level greater than 99% between sex and EOP.

The strength of the association can be measured by Cramer's V^2 which is a modification of a ϕ^2 measure of association. ϕ^2 is simply the calculated value of χ^2 divided by the total sample size. Thus, $\phi^2 = 492.7/1000 \approx 0.49$. To calculate Cramer's V^2 we simply divide this by the minimum of the number of rows -1, or number of columns -1. There are two columns and three rows, therefore the number of columns -1, which equals 1 is the appropriate divisor. As $0.49/1 = 0.49$. This is a measure association between EOP and sex in the Anatolian sample.

There is a significant association between sex and EOP, and a reasonably high strength of association. By inspection of the table above it can be seen that type I EOP is mostly a female trait, type III mostly a male trait, and type II not related to either sex. Gülekon and Turgut (2003) concluded that EOP would be a good property to consider to estimate the sex of an unknown individual, and from the analysis above this view is justifiable.

Solutions to Chapter 6

1. The linear correlation coefficients are:

(a) 0.71
(b) 0.95
(c) −0.12
(d) 0.23
(e) −0.55
(f) −0.01
(g) −0.76
(h) −0.96
(i) 0.50

2. A plot of the first 10 points of data from Levine *et al.* (2002, Table 1) is below:

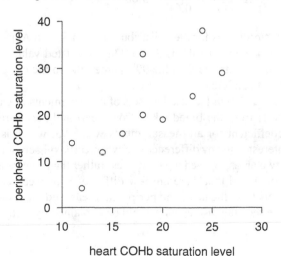

From the scatterplot we might expect a reasonably high linear correlation between the carboxyhaemoglobin saturation levels from the blood taken from heart and peripheral areas.

COHb heart	$x - \bar{x}$	$(x - \bar{x})^2$	COHb peripheral	$y - \bar{y}$	$(y - \bar{y})^2$	$(x - \bar{x})(y - \bar{y})$
11	−7.2	51.84	14	−6.92	47.89	49.82
12	−6.2	38.44	4.2	−16.72	279.56	103.66
14	−4.2	17.64	12	−8.92	79.57	37.46
16	−2.2	4.84	16	−4.92	24.21	10.82
18	−0.2	0.04	20	−0.92	0.85	0.18
18	−0.2	0.04	33	12.08	145.93	−2.42
20	1.8	3.24	19	−1.92	3.69	−3.46
23	4.8	23.04	24	3.08	9.49	14.78
24	5.8	33.64	38	17.08	291.73	99.06
26	7.8	60.84	29	8.08	65.29	63.02
$\bar{x} = 18.20$		$\sum 233.60$	$\bar{y} = 20.92$		$\sum 948.18$	$\sum 372.96$

Using values from the table the correlation coefficient r from Equation 12 on p. 57 is equal to:

$$\frac{372.96}{\sqrt{233.60 \times 948.18}} = \frac{372.96}{470.63} = 0.79$$

which is a high linear correlation between carboxyhaemoglobin saturation levels from the blood taken from heart and peripheral areas in this sample.

A test statistic is given in Equation 13 on p. 59. We have 10 xy pairs, thus 8 df, so the value of the test statistic is:

$$t = \frac{0.79 \times \sqrt{8}}{\sqrt{1 - 0.79^2}} = \frac{2.23}{0.61} = 3.66$$

Looking up the ordinates for the t-distribution with 8 df in Appendix C we find that at 99% confidence a value of t is 3.355. Our calculated value of 3.66 exceeds this value, thus is more extreme than the 99th percentile, so the correlation is significant at a high level of confidence.

Levine *et al.* (2002) in fact used 42 sets of measurements of carboxyhaemoglobin saturation levels from the blood taken from heart and peripheral areas. The linear correlation coefficient for all measurements was 0.93, which is very high. Levine *et al.* were interested in any differences between carboxyhaemoglobin saturation levels from the two areas, so used a paired t-test rather than a correlation test illustrated here. They concluded that there are few differences between carboxyhaemoglobin saturation levels from the heart and peripheral areas, and the few cases where differences could be seen the discrepancy could be explained by factors such as acuteness of death.

3. The correlation matrix from the question is reproduced here. The variables are age in years, D/L ratio of aspartic acid and D/L ratio of glutamic acid measured from the acid-insoluble, collagen-rich fraction from the femur in 21 cadivars of known age at death.

	age	aspartic	glutamic
age	1.00	0.97	0.88
aspartic	–	1.00	0.86
glutamic	–	–	1.00

Ohtani *et al.* (2004) claimed that the D/L ratio of aspartic acid is the best of the measured amino acid ratios for age estimation. With a correlation coefficient of 0.97 for aspartic acid against a correlation coefficient of 0.88 for glutamic acid this would appear to be the case, but is it really so much better?

We notice that D/L ratio of aspartic is also heavily correlated with the D/L ratio of glutamic acid, so it is unlikely that the correlation coefficients of 0.97 and 0.88 represent the true strength of the D/L ratios of the respective amino acids with age. It would be useful to know the partial correlation coefficients for these variables.

Turning to Equation 14 on p. 67 we see that:

$$r_{ij\,|k} = \frac{r_{ij} - r_{ik}\,r_{jk}}{\sqrt{1 - r_{ik}^2}\sqrt{1 - r_{jk}^2}}$$

If we call age $= i$, aspartic $= j$ and glutamic $= k$, then the partial correlation between age and aspartic acid controlling for the effects of the correlation with glutamic acid is:

$$r_{ij\,|k} = \frac{0.97 - (0.88 \times 0.86)}{\sqrt{1 - 0.88^2}\sqrt{1 - 0.86^2}} = \frac{0.2132}{0.4749 \times 0.5103} = 0.8798 \approx 0.88$$

Now let aspartic $= i$, glutamic $= j$ and age $= k$, then the partial correlation between aspartic acid and glutamic acid controlling for the effects of the correlation with age:

$$r_{ij\,|k} = \frac{0.86 - (0.97 \times 0.88)}{\sqrt{1 - 0.97^2}\sqrt{1 - 0.88^2}} = \frac{0.0064}{0.2431 \times 0.4749} = 0.0554 \approx 0.06$$

And finally, let age $= i$, glutamic $= j$, and aspartic $= k$, so that the partial correlation between age and glutamic acid controlling for the effects of aspartic acid is:

$$r_{ij\,|k} = \frac{0.88 - (0.97 \times 0.86)}{\sqrt{1 - 0.97^2}\sqrt{1 - 0.86^2}} = \frac{0.0458}{0.2431 \times 0.5103} = 0.3692 \approx 0.37$$

We can now enter the partial correlation coefficients into a table:

	age	aspartic	glutamic
age	1.00	0.88	0.37
aspartic	–	1.00	0.06
glutamic	–	–	1.00

The partial correlation table suggests that D/L glutamic acid ratios and D/L aspartic acid ratios are not linearly related when the effects of age are controlled for. This is expected as aspartic acid and glutamic acid should not affect each other's rate of racemization. More importantly the partial correlation coefficient between age and glutamic acid is only 0.37, a value for t calculated from Equation 13 on p. 59 using $21 - 3 = 18$ df is $t = 1.689$, which from the table in Appendix C is smaller than the value of 2.101, indicating that the partial linear correlation is not significant at the 95% confidence. The partial correlation coefficient of 0.88 for aspartic acid and age is significant at the 1% level ($t = 7.86$). Therefore, when Ohtani *et al.* (2004) claim that the D/L ratio of aspartic acid is the best indicator of age they are absolutely correct, as the D/L ratio of glutamic hardly correlated with age when the effect of the correlation with aspartic acid is taken into account.

Solutions to Chapter 7

1. The data provided by Scott and Oliver (2001) contain elements which are 'not detected'. It is difficult to know whether these are true zeros, that is, diazepam is not there, or something is amiss with the detection aparatus. Scott and Oliver (2001) treated the not detected values as true zeros, so obviously these were simply below minimum detectable level. As we are calculating by hand it will be expedient to disregard observations where one, or both, observations are not detected.

Here are their results with the 'not detected' values removed:

Vitreous humor (mg/l)	Blood (mg/l)
1.98	0.63
0.44	0.39
1.01	0.74
0.47	0.47
0.15	0.15
0.45	0.07
0.03	0.01
0.27	0.10
0.08	0.10
1.51	1.25
2.62	2.48

Scott and Oliver (2001) say that 'The transport of drugs across the blood vitreous humor barrier is limited by the lipid solubility of . . .'.

This is a clear piece of background theory which informs us which way round the model should be fitted. In this instance diazepam in the blood is transferred through some mechanism to the vitreous humor, so blood diazepam can be said to 'cause' vitreous humor. The correct way to fit these data is to fit vitreous humor diazepam concentration (y) to blood diazepam concentration (x).

Here is a graph of these data.

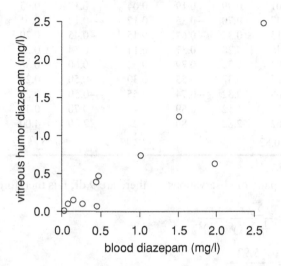

From inspection of the graph the relationship looks linear.

x	$x - \bar{x}$	$(x - \bar{x})^2$	y	$y - \bar{y}$	$(x - \bar{x})(y - \bar{y})$
0.63	0.05	0.00	1.98	1.16	0.06
0.39	−0.19	0.04	0.44	−0.38	0.07
0.74	0.16	0.03	1.01	0.19	0.03
0.47	−0.11	0.01	0.47	−0.35	0.04
0.15	−0.43	0.18	0.15	−0.67	0.29
0.07	−0.51	0.26	0.45	−0.37	0.19
0.01	−0.57	0.32	0.03	−0.79	0.45
0.10	−0.48	0.23	0.27	−0.55	0.26
0.10	−0.48	0.23	0.08	−0.74	0.36
1.25	0.67	0.45	1.51	0.69	0.46
2.48	1.90	3.61	2.62	1.80	3.42
$\bar{x} = 0.58$		$\sum 5.36$	$\bar{y} = 0.82$		$\sum 5.63$

From the table $S_{xx} = 5.36$ and $S_{xy} = 5.63$ so $b = 1.05$. From the table $\bar{x} = 0.58$ and $\bar{y} = 0.82$, therefore $a = 0.82 - (0.58 \times 1.05) = 0.21$.

Now that we have calculated b and a estimates for vitreous humor ($\hat{y}$) can be made, as can goodness of fit statistics.

x	y	$\hat{y}$	$y - \bar{y}$	$(y - \bar{y})^2$	$\hat{y} - \bar{y}$	$(\hat{y} - \bar{y})^2$	$y - \hat{y}$	$(y - \hat{y})^2$
0.63	1.98	0.87	1.16	1.35	0.05	0.00	1.11	1.23
0.39	0.44	0.62	−0.38	0.14	−0.20	0.04	−0.18	0.03
0.74	1.01	0.99	0.19	0.04	0.17	0.03	0.02	0.00
0.47	0.47	0.70	−0.35	0.12	−0.12	0.01	−0.23	0.05
0.15	0.15	0.37	−0.67	0.45	−0.45	0.20	−0.22	0.05
0.07	0.45	0.28	−0.37	0.14	−0.54	0.29	0.17	0.03
0.01	0.03	0.22	−0.79	0.62	−0.60	0.36	−0.19	0.04
0.10	0.27	0.32	−0.55	0.30	−0.50	0.25	−0.05	0.00
0.10	0.08	0.32	−0.74	0.55	−0.50	0.25	−0.24	0.06
1.25	1.51	1.52	0.69	0.48	0.70	0.49	−0.01	0.00
2.48	2.62	2.82	1.80	3.24	2.00	4.00	−0.2	0.04
$\bar{x} = 0.58$	$\bar{y} = 0.82$			$\sum 7.43$		$\sum 5.92$		$\sum 1.53$

There are 11 pairs of observations, so there are 9 df; F is therefore:

$$F = \frac{\sum(\hat{y} - \bar{y})^2}{\frac{1}{df}\sum(y - \hat{y})^2}$$

$$= \frac{5.92}{\frac{1}{9} \times 1.53}$$

$$= \frac{5.92}{0.17}$$

$$= 34.82$$

From Appendix F the value of F at the 1% level is 10.56. The calculated value of F from the regression is 34.82, which means that the calculated value of F is more extreme than the value of F at 1%, so there is reason to think that the model is a good fit to these data.

The residual plot for this model is:

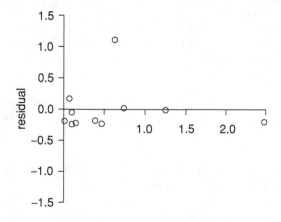

blood diazepam (mg/l)

and with the exception of one point the residual plot gives no indication that the model violates any regression assumption.

Scott and Oliver (2001) suggest that the regression coefficient b is different from 1. The value of b from the fit of vitreous humor diazepam concentration is 1.05, however, the standard error for b is:

$$ESE(b) = \frac{s}{\sqrt{S_{xx}}}$$

where:

$$s^2 = \frac{S_{yy} - \frac{S_{xy}^2}{S_{xx}}}{n-2}$$

$S_{yy} = \sum(y - \bar{y})^2 = 7.43$ from the table above. $S_{xy} = \sum(x - \bar{x})(y - \bar{y}) = 5.63$, and $S_{xx} = \sum(x - \bar{x})^2 = 5.36$, giving

$$s^2 = \frac{7.43 - \frac{5.63^2}{5.36}}{9}$$

$$= \frac{7.43 - \frac{31.70}{5.36}}{9}$$

$$= \frac{7.43 - 5.91}{9}$$

$$= \frac{7.43 - 5.91}{9}$$

$$= 0.17$$

Therefore $s = 0.41$ and $ESE(b) = 0.41/5.36 = 0.076$. From Appendix D for 9 df, $t = 2.262$, thus a suitable 95% confidence interval for b is $1.05 \pm 2.262 \times 0.076$, which gives a 95% confidence interval for b from 0.88 to 1.22. This interval includes 1, so at 95% confidence there is no reason to reject 1 as a possible value for b.

Scott and Oliver (2001) fitted blood diazepam concentration to vitreous humor concentration. This gave a gradient b of 0.72 with a standard error of 0.044. A 95% confidence interval would not have contained 1 as a possible value for b.

Scott and Oliver (2001) give no particular reason for fitting blood diazepam concentration to vitreous humor diazepam concentration. As the production of a calibration model for blood diazepam concentration from vitreous humor diazepam concentration was not one of their objectives, the direction of fitting makes no great difference to their conclusions.

2. We need to work out a point estimate and confidence interval for age of the offender when the tooth was extracted using the data supplied by Gillard *et al.* (1990). First we need to work out which way round any linear model needs to be fitted. Time can be said to cause change in the %D-aspartic acid, so age will be x, and %D-aspartic acid will be y.

The accompanying summary statistics are replicated here:

$\bar{x}$	29.73
$\bar{y}$	2.06
$\sum(x - \bar{x})(y - \bar{y})$	268.03
$\sum(x - \bar{x})^2$	5390.15
$\sum(\hat{y} - \bar{x})^2$	13.28
$\sum(y - \hat{x})^2$	0.54

Here is a plot of the two covariates:

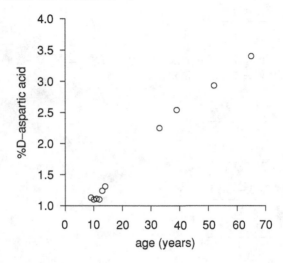

In the xy plot there is some hint of non-linearity which is a very small effect, and could be due to the fact that from background theory %D-aspartic acid is not quite linear (Ohtani *et al.*, 2004). As we are only given %D-aspartic acid we cannot calculate $(1 + D/L)/(1 - D/L)$ to obtain theoretically linear data. Looking at a 'goodness of fit' statistic F:

$$F = \frac{\sum(\hat{y} - \bar{y})^2}{\frac{1}{df}\sum(y - \hat{y})^2}$$

$$= \frac{13.28}{\frac{1}{9} \times 0.54}$$

$$= 221.33$$

From Appendix F, for 9 df, F = 5.12 at 95% confidence, and 10.56 at 99% confidence. The calculated value of F is more extreme than either of these values, so there is unlikely to be any 'lack of fit' between the data and linear model.

We know that:

$$b = \frac{S_{xy}}{S_{xx}} = \frac{\sum(x - \bar{x})(y - \bar{y})}{\sum(x - \bar{x})^2} = \frac{268.03}{5390.15} = 0.0497$$

and:

$$a = \bar{y} - b\bar{x} = 2.06 - (0.0497 \times 29.73) = 0.58$$

With a model we can now calculate estimates for %D-aspartic acid and examine a residual plot:

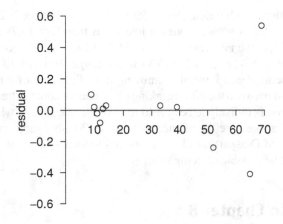

age (years)

The residuals look slightly heteroscedastic. The clump of low value points look as though they could be autocorrelated, although there is no mechanism which would allow this unless the study of Gillard *et al.* (1990) used longitudinal data which they do not mention. There are, however, very few points in this reduced dataset, so what we see in the residual plot may just be an artifact of these particular data.

The %D-aspartic acid from the offender is 2.01, so the point estimate of the offender's age is:

$$x_0 = \frac{2.06 - 0.58}{0.0497} = 29.78$$

The standard error $S_{x/y}$ is:

$$S_{y/x} = \sqrt{\frac{\sum(y - \hat{y})^2}{n - 2}}$$

In this case $S_{y/x} = \sqrt{0.54/9} = \sqrt{0.06} = 0.24$. The standard error associated with the estimate of x is:

$$S_{x0} = \frac{S_{y/x}}{b} \sqrt{\left\{ 1 + \frac{1}{n} + \frac{(y_0 - \bar{y})^2}{b^2 \sum(x - \bar{x})^2} \right\}}$$

$$= \frac{0.24}{0.0497} \sqrt{\left\{ 1 + \frac{1}{11} + \frac{(2.01 - 2.06)^2}{0.0497^2 \times 5391.15)^2} \right\}}$$

$$= 4.829\sqrt{1 + \frac{1}{11} + \frac{-0.05^2}{0.0025 \times 5390.15}}$$

$$= 4.829\sqrt{1.091}$$

$$= 5.04$$

From Appendix C with 9 df the value for t at 95% confidence is 2.262, at 99% confidence $t = 3.250$. A 95% confidence interval is therefore $29.78 \pm 2.262 \times 5.04 = 29.78 \pm 11.40$ so the interval is 18.38 to 41.18 years. A 99% confidence interval is $29.78 \pm 3.250 \times 5.04 = 29.78 \pm 16.38$ which ranges from 13.40 to 46.16 years.

Given the confidence intervals, removing the adjustment of 9 months to account for the interval between the offence taking place and the tooth extracted is immaterial. This calibration is unlikely to be able to resolve the question of whether the offender was 21 or 22 at the time the offence took place. Possibly more modern methods of measurement of D-aspartic and L-aspartic acids such as presented by Ohtani *et al.* (2004) might be capable of doing so.

Solutions to Chapter 8

1. Silver is a very common colour for the Ford Focuss. The silver paint which could not be excluded by the examiner occurs on many other cars, both Focusses and others in the Ford range. Despite being very sure that the paint is the same *type* of paint as that used in Focusses the evidence is not terribly persuasive.

2. Vivid lime green is not a very common colour for anything, let alone cars. There are very few vehicles with this type of paint, so the evidence is more persuasive.

Solutions to Chapter 9

1. The data for the location of gunshot wounds by mode of death is replicated here with row and column sums appended:

	homicide	suicide	Σ
skull	33	34	67
spine	16	1	17
torso	29	13	42
limbs	12	1	13
Σ	90	49	139

Denote the area in which gunshot wounds from the sample have been located as l, with suffixes sk, sp, to, lg to indicate the specific area, so l_{sp} would indicate a gunshot wound to the spine. Denote the mode of death as d with suffixes h and s to indicate homicide and suicide respectively, so d_s indicates suicide.

(a) Of 139 individuals in the sample 90 were homicides, so $Pr(d_h) = 90/139 = 0.647$, or 64.7%

(b) The number of individuals who committed suicide *and* had a gunshot wound to the torso is 13. In notation this is $Pr(d_s, l_{to})$ which is the probability of the joint event torso, and suicide. There are 139 individuals in total, therefore the probability of finding both wound to torso and suicide is $13/139 = 0.093 \approx 9\%$

(c) We are asked to calculate a value for $Pr(l_{sp} \mid d_h)$. As we know the mode of death we need only concern ourselves with the left-hand column. In the sample 90 individuals have been subjected to homicide, of whom 16 display gunshot wounds to the spine. Thus $Pr(l_{sp} \mid d_h) = 16/90 = 0.178$, or nearly 18%.

(d) This asks for $Pr(d_h \mid l_{sp})$. As the wound is in the spine we need only consider the second row. From the table, 17 individuals have gunshot wounds to the spine, and of those 16 were homicides. $Pr(d_h \mid l_{sp}) = 16/17 = 0.941 \approx 94\%$, therefore there is a 94% probability that an individual from the sample who had a gunshot wound to the spine was a homicide.

Notice the contrast in the figures here between 18% and 94% in what verbally sound like very similar propositions.

(e) We are asked for $Pr(d_s \mid l_{lg})$. As we know the wound was to the left leg, and that the left leg is a limb, we are only really concerned with the fourth row of data in the table which refers to wounds to the limbs. The total number of individuals with wounds to the limbs is 13, one of whom committed suicide. Therefore $Pr(d_s \mid l_{lg}) = 1/13 = 0.076$, which $\approx 7\%$.

(f) This time we need $Pr(l_{lg} \mid d_s)$ as the left leg is a limb, and the question asks for the left leg. From the sample 49 individuals committed suicide, of whom one had a gunshot wound to the limbs. That means $Pr(l_{lg} \mid d_s) = 1/49 = 0.020 = 2\%$. However, as the left leg is only one of four possible limbs, and the question instructs us to treat each limb as equally likely to be wounded, $Pr(l_{\text{left leg}} \mid d_s) = 0.020/4 = 0.005$ or 0.5%.

Again notice the difference in results for what sound like similar propositions.

2. The most general form of Bayes' theorem is given in Equation 22 on p. 109 and is reproduced here:

$$Pr(H \mid E) = \frac{Pr(E \mid H) \times Pr(H)}{Pr(E)}$$

Denote C as a proposition, H as homicide and S as suicide. From the question $C = \{H, S\}$. Denote W as wound, where $W = \{Sk, Sp, To, Li\}$, where Sk is skull, Sp is spine, To torso, and Li limbs.

De la Grandmaison *et al.*'s (2001) data is reproduced here:

	homicide	suicide	$\sum$
skull	33	34	67
spine	16	1	17
torso	29	13	42
limbs	12	1	13
$\sum$	90	49	139

and from the question there are 1500 suicides, and 800 homicides a year in the United Kingdom. So: $Pr(S) = 1500/(1500 + 800) = 15/23$ and $Pr(H) = 800/(1500 + 800) = 8/23$. The question this time does not state that victim is drawn the from the sample. It is a matter for debat, but a more suitable set of prior probabilities may be those for homicides and suicides for the UK as s whole, rather than the sample.

Restating Bayes' theorem we can say:

$$Pr(C \mid W) = \frac{Pr(W \mid C) \times Pr(C)}{Pr(W \mid H) \times Pr(H) + Pr(W \mid S) \times Pr(S)}$$

(a) As the wound in this case is to the left leg, and the left leg is a limb we will look at row 4 in the table. From this we can say: $Pr(Li \mid H) = 12/90$, and $Pr(Li \mid S) = 1/49$. Substituting these values into the equation above:

$$Pr(H \mid Li) = \frac{12/90 \times 8/23}{(12/90 \times 8/23) + (1/49 \times 15/23)}$$

$$= \frac{96/2070}{96/2070 + 15/1127}$$

$$= 0.777$$

or, there is an 77.7% probability that a body observed with gunshot wounds to its leg was the result of a homicide.

(b) This question is very similar to the one above, but this time the question asks about wounds to the head. The prior probabilities remain the same, only the likelihoods change.

In this case we want $Pr(Sk \mid H)$ and $Pr(Sk \mid S)$ which, as the skull may be thought of as the head, are from row 1 of the table $Pr(Sk \mid H) = 33/90$, and $Pr(Sk \mid S) = 34/49$. Substituting these into the equation above:

$$Pr(H \mid Li) = \frac{33/90 \times 8/23}{(33/90 \times 8/23) + (34/49 \times 15/23)}$$

$$= \frac{264/2070}{264/2070 + 510/1127}$$

$$= 0.219$$

or a 22% probability that an individual committed suicide upon the observation of a gunshot wound to the head.

(c) This is a trick question. It asks whether, given someone has committed suicide, what is the probability they have a gunshot wound to the torso. We know from the question that given a gunshot wound, the only possible means of death would be homicide and suicide, but given suicide we know nothing about the other possible means of death. What we would need to answer this question is the proportion of suicides who shoot themselves.

Solutions to Chapter 13

1. (a) *There is a 1% chance of observing the blood type were the defendant innocent, therefore there is a 99% probability the defendent is guilty.*

 The data tell us that there is a 1% *chance of observing the DNA profile were the defendant innocent*. This corresponds to $\Pr(E \mid \overline{G})$. The conclusion is that *there is a 99% probability the defendant is guilty,* which is $\Pr(G \mid E)$. This is a transposition of the conditional from the data.

(b) *From binomial theorem there is a 99% probability that there are over* 10 000 *individuals in the United Kingdom with this blood type. Therefore the evidence is useless as there is only a* 1/10 000 *probability the suspect is guilty.*

 As there are in excess of 10 000 individuals in the United Kingdom, population 60 000 000, the evidence is potentially of quite some probative value as it narrows the potential pool of suspects from 60 000 000 to 10 000. The statement makes the defender's fallacy by suggesting the evidence is of little probative value. It is true that if the offender has to be one of the 10 000 individuals with the blood group, all of whom were equally likely to be guilty, there would be a 1/10 000 probability the suspect was guilty. However, this assessment would not evaluate the evidence, but would seek to comment upon the *ultimate issue*.

(c) *The evidence of a DNA match is* 10 000 *times as likely were the DNA profile to have come from the suspect as some other individual in the population. Therefore the blood is* 10 000 *times more likely to have come from the suspect than from someone else.*

 Here we are provided with a likelihood ratio for the evidence, which is the observation of a match. In the conclusions this has been transposed to the likelihood ratio for the source of the blood, which is not the same thing at all. Basically this conclusion cannot be drawn from the likelihood ratio as they address different questions.

2. There are two errors of interpretation.

(a) The paint flecks match with a probability of 99% by colour and composition, which, with no mention of any background database means confidence about distributional means is being misappropriated to stand in for a probability that the two paints are in fact the same paint, thus committing the *different level* error.

(b) Even if it were true that there is a 99% probability that the paint from the first car matches that from the second, this is far from saying the cars were involved in a collision; a more correct statement would be that there is a 99% probability that the second car was the source of the paint on the first car. This is an error where the scientist has attempted to draw conclusions about the activities of the two cars, rather than simply commenting on the source of paint flecks.

3. The distribution in Table 3.3 on p. 26 gives $Pr(T \mid Y)$, where T is THC content, and Y is year. In the case of Table 3.3 the year is restricted to 1986. To make an assignment of year (Y) based on THC contect (T) would require $Pr(Y \mid T)$, which is not given in the table. So the error is one of the *transposed conditional*, or, *prosecutor's fallacy*.

Solutions to Chapter 14

1. To recap: *use Table 14.1 to calculate a value of evidence from the allelic frequencies for LDLR(A, A), GYPA(A, B), HBGG(B, B), D7S8(A, B) and Gc(A, C).*

    First we need to know the allelic frequencies. This can be calculated from the genotype frequencies given in Table 14.1 on p. 163 using Equation 33 reproduced here:

$$P_i = P_{ii} + \frac{1}{2} \sum_{i \neq j}^{n} P_{ij}$$

    For LDLR we only need to find P_a which is $P_a = 0.127 + \frac{1}{2}(0.503) = 0.378$.

    For GYPA we need to know both P_a and P_b. $P_a = 0.306 + \frac{1}{2}(0.522) = 0.567$, and $P_b = 0.172 + \frac{1}{2}(0.522) = 0.433$.

    HBGG we need P_b which is given by $P_b = 0.306 + \frac{1}{2}(0.553 + 0.00) = 0.582$.

    S7S8 we need P_a and P_b: $P_a = 0.382 + \frac{1}{2}(0.522) = 0.643$, and $P_b = 0.096 + \frac{1}{2}(0.522) = 0.357$.

    For Gc again we need both P_a and P_b: $P_a = 0.064 + \frac{1}{2}(0.083 + 0.306) = 0.258$, and $P_b = 0.343 + \frac{1}{2}(0.306 + 0.159) = 0.575$.

    Using Equation 34 (reproduced here):

$$\left. \begin{array}{l} Pr_{ii} = Pr_i^2 \\ Pr_{ij} = 2 Pr_i Pr_j, \ j \neq i \end{array} \right\}$$

    If linkage equllibrium can be assumed, the probability of this particular genetic profile is therefore: $0.378^2 \times 2(0.567 \times 0.172) \times 0.582^2 \times 2(0.643 \times 0.357) \times 2(0.258 \times 0.575)$ which is ≈ 0.0013, so the value is ≈ 777 given a match.

2. The value from the genotypic frequencies was calculated in Section 14.2 p. 162, and was 594, which is smaller than the value using Hardy-Weinberg equilibrium as an assumption, which from above was 777. In this case the assumption of Hardy-Weinberg equilibrium has favoured the prosecution.

3. Ülküer *et al.* (1999) specifically state that they suspected the HBGG locus as not conforming to Hardy-Weinberg conditions, which is one of the reasons they published the genotype data. The genotype frequency for HBGG(B, B) from Ülküer *et al.* (1999) is 0.306, from the allelic frequencies above HBGG(B, B) occurs with a frequency 0.339, which is actually greater than the observed frequency, so cannot be the source of the error favouring the prosecution. If the observed frequency is employed rather than the calculated frequency for HBGG(B, B) the value is ≈ 860. It is left as a longer term exercise to find where the discrepancy between the two values lies.

4. Equation 35 on p. 168 is appropriate:

$$\left. \begin{array}{l} Pr_{ii} = \dfrac{[2F + (1 - F)p_i][3F + (1 - F)p_i]}{(1 + F)(1 + 2F)} \\[2ex] Pr_{ij} = \dfrac{2[F + (1 - F)p_i][F + (1 - F)p_j]}{(1 + F)(1 + 2F)} \end{array} \right\}$$

Using the allelic frequencies calculated above the genotype proportions are: $P_{\text{LDLR}(A,A)} = 0.178$, $P_{\text{GYPA}(A,B)} = 0.104$, $P_{\text{HBGG}(B,B)} = 0.374$, $P_{\text{G7S8}(A,B)} = 0.225$, $P_{\text{Gc}(A,C)} = 0.151$. If linkage equilibrium can be assumed then the probability of finding the profile in the population is ≈ 0.000235 which gives a value of 4251.

Solutions to Chapter 15

1. Reproducing the table in the question:

Locus	G_c	G_m	G_{pp}
TPOX	(6, 6)	(9, 6)	(12, 6)
VWA	(18, 21)	(16, 21)	(18, 21)
THO1	(9, 9.3)	(6, 9.3)	(9, 10)

At TPOX $G_c(6, 6)$, $G_m(9, 6)$ and $G_{pp}(12, 6)$. If $i = 6$, $j = 9$ and $k = 12$ this is the same situation as in row 6 of Table 15.1 on p. 174. $LR(G_c \mid G_{pp}) = \frac{1}{2p_i}$. i in this instance is allele 6, which, from Table 14.3, occurs with frequency 0.006, hence the contribution to the likelihood ratio is $\frac{1}{0.012} = 83.33$.

At VWA $G_c(18, 21)$, $G_m(16, 21)$ and $G_{pp}(18, 21)$. Let $i = 21$, $j = 18$ and $k = 16$. The position is the same as the fourth row from bottom in Table 15.1 so that the likelihood ratio is $\frac{1}{2p_j}$. $j = 18$ which occurs in the Turkish population with relative frequency 0.205 from Table 14.3. So $LR(G_c \mid G_{pp}) = \frac{1}{2 \times 0.205} = 2.44$.

The profiles at the THO1 locus are $G_c(9, 9.3)$, $G_m(6, 9.3)$ and $G_{pp}(9, 10)$. If $i = 9.3$, $j = 9$, $k = 6$ and $l = 10$, then the situation is the same as the second row from the bottom on Table 15.1, so that the likelihood ratio is $\frac{1}{2p_j}$ as $j = 9$, which from Table 14.3 occurs with relative frequency 0.232 in the Turkish population. So $LR(G_c \mid G_{pp}) = \frac{1}{2 \times 0.232} = 2.16$.

As linkage equilibrium can be assumed the likelihood ratio for the whole profile is the product of the likelihood ratios for the individual loci, so $LR(G_c \mid G_{pp}) = 83.33 \times 2.44 \times 2.16 = 439.18 \approx 439$. The value of the profile in this instance is that it ≈ 439 times more likely if $G_{pp} = G_p$ than if $G_{pp} \neq G_p$.

2. Reproducing the table from the question:

Locus	G_c	G_m	G_{pp}
TPOX	(6, 6)	(9, 6)	(12, 6)
VWA	(18, 21)	(16, 21)	(18, 21)
THO1	(9, 9.3)	(6, 9.3)	(8, 10)

If the putative paternal profile is examined at the THO1 locus it will be noticed that he possesses alleles 8 and 10, the child has alleles 9 and 9.3, hence this man cannot be the father of this child as the two have no common alleles.

3. Reproducing the table from the question:

Locus	G_c	G_m	G_{pp}
LDLR	(A, B)	(A, B)	(B, B)
GYPA	(A, B)	(A, A)	(B, B)
HBGG	(B, B)	(B, B)	(B, B)
D7S8	(A, B)	(A, B)	(A, B)
Gc	(A, C)	(A, B)	(B, C)

For the LDLR locus $G_c(A, B)$ while $G_m(A, B)$ and $G_{pp}(B, B)$. Let $A = j$, and $B = i$, this corresponds to the 12th row of Table 15.1 . As both linkage and Hardy-Weinberg eqilibrium may be assumed then $LR(G_c \mid G_{pp}) = \frac{1}{p_i+p_j}$.

If $A = i$ and $B = j$ for the GYPA locus then from the 8th row of Table 15.1 $LR(G_c \mid G_{pp}) = \frac{1}{p_j}$.

If $B = i$ for HBGG then the first row of Table 15.1 gives $LR(G_c \mid G_{pp}) = \frac{1}{p_i}$.

For D7S8 let $A = i$ and $B = j$ the 13th row of Table 15.1 gives $LR(G_c \mid G_{pp}) = \frac{1}{p_i+p_j}$.

If $A = i$, $C = j$ and $B = k$ for Gc, then the third row from the bottom of Table 15.1 gives $LR(G_c \mid G_{pp}) = \frac{1}{2p_j}$.

From Table 14.1 we know LDLR(A, A) occurs with relative frequency 0.127, and LDLR(A, B) occurs with frequency 0.503. From Equation 33:

$$P_i = P_{ii} + \frac{1}{2} \sum_{i \neq j}^{n} P_{ij}$$

so the allele LDLR(A) occurs with frequency $0.127 + (0.503/2) = 0.378$.

Applying the same reasoning the relative frequency for LDLR(B) is 0.622. Thus $LR(G_c \mid G_{pp}) = \frac{1}{0.378+0.622} = 1$. This result is expected as the likelihood ratio is the reciprocal of the sum of the relative frequencies of the two alleles. As there are only two alleles for LDLR the sum of their relative frequencies must be one, making the likelihood ratio also equal to one.

For locus GYPA we need only calculate the relative frequency of the B allele. From Table 14.1 allele B occurs $0.306 + (0.522/2) = 0.567$. So $LR(G_c \mid G_{pp}) = \frac{1}{0.567} = 1.763$.

We also need only calculate the relative frequency of the HBGG allele B, which from Table 14.1 is $0.306 + (0.573/2) = 0.592$, so $LR(G_c \mid G_{pp}) = \frac{1}{0.592} = 1.687$.

For D7S8 the relative frequencies of alleles A and B must be calculated. But from Table 14.1 we know there are only two alleles at D7S8, and from above the $LR(G_c \mid G_{pp}) = \frac{1}{p_i+p_j}$, which is the same situation as for locus LDLR. So $LR(G_c \mid G_{pp}) = 1$.

With Gc we need only calculate the relative frequency of allele C, which from Table 14.1 is $0.343 + \frac{1}{2}(0.159 + 0.306) = 0.575$. The likelihood ratio for Gc is $\frac{1}{2}(p_j)$ which in this case is $1/1.151 = 0.869$.

As linkage equilibruum can be assumed the evidential value for the match is the product of all the individual likelihood ratios, which is $1 \times 1.763 \times 1.687 \times 1 \times$

$0.869 = 2.585$, which means that the match is ≈ 2.5 times as likely were $G_{pp} = G_p$ than $G_{pp} \neq G_p$.

Solutions to Chapter 16

1. From Equation 7 on p. 31:

$$\text{standard error of the mean } (x) = \frac{\text{sd}}{\sqrt{n}}$$

From the table in Appendix B we know that at 99% confidence we need to leave 0.005% of the distribution in *each* tail, so the ordinate which corresponds 0.995% of the area under the curve is 2.58. As 100 g is 2.58 standard errors we can set a single standard error to $100/2.58 = 38.76$ g. So:

$$38.76 = \frac{240}{\sqrt{n}}$$

$$38.76\sqrt{n} = 240$$

$$\sqrt{n} = \frac{240}{38.76}$$

$$\sqrt{n} = 6.16$$

$$n = 38.34$$

Rounding up we would require 39 measurements of victims of SIDS brain weights to be 99% confident that the mean was known to ± 100 g.

2. Summarizing the data from Thompson and Cohle (2004) on the brain weights of SIDS and non-SIDS infants:

	SIDS	non-SIDS
mean brain weight (g)	953	905
standard deviation (g)	240	238
sample size	5	7

The standardized distance δ is calculated from:

$$\delta = \frac{\text{difference}}{2 \times \sqrt{\text{pooled variance}}}$$

where an estimate of the pooled variance is given by Equations 9 on p. 37. This is:

$$\hat{s} = \sqrt{\frac{(n_1 - 1)s_1^2 + (n_2 - 1)s_2^2}{n_1 + n_2 - 2}}$$

As the variance is the square of the standard deviation s_1^2 is 57600 and s_2^2 is 56644, $n_1 = 5$ and $n_2 = 7$ then an estimate of the pooled variance is:

$$\hat{s} = \sqrt{\frac{(4 \times 57600) + (6 \times 56644)}{5 + 7 - 2}}$$

$$= \sqrt{\frac{288000 + 396508}{10}}$$

$$= \sqrt{68450.8}$$

$$= 261.63$$

The difference between the two means of brain weights is $953 - 905 = 48\,\text{g}$ so:

$$\delta = \frac{48}{2 \times \sqrt{261.63}}$$

$$= \frac{48}{2 \times 16.18}$$

$$= 1.48$$

Inspection of the operating characteristic curve (Figure 16.1 would indicate that the probability of making a Type II error (not detecting an difference when a difference is in fact true) is 0.10 for $n = 10$, and 0.05 for $n = 12$ for $\delta = 1.5$. As in the original work by Thompson and Cohle (2004) n was equal to 12. This means that the probability of making a Type II error was 0.05, and that their sample size was perfectly adequate for differences observed between SIDS and non-SIDS infants.

3. From the consignment ten sub-units have been examined and nine found to contain cocaine. If a uniform distribution is considered appropriate for the prior knowledge of the proportion of positive units in the consignment, then by looking up row 9 for one negative at 99% probability in the table in Appendix E we see that at least 0.53 of the consignment contain cocaine. 53% of 348 sub-units is 194.88 sub-units, or 194 sub-units. So we can be 99% sure that at least 194 sub-units are positive for cocaine.

Appendix B
Percentage points of the standard normal distribution

Probability α under curve to z. For negative z use $1 - \alpha$.
   So probability α at $z = -2$ is 0.0228.

z	0.00	0.01	0.02	0.03	0.04	0.05	0.06	0.07	0.08	0.09
0.0	0.5000	0.5040	0.5080	0.5120	0.5160	0.5199	0.5239	0.5279	0.5319	0.5359
0.1	0.5398	0.5438	0.5478	0.5517	0.5557	0.5596	0.5636	0.5675	0.5714	0.5753
0.2	0.5793	0.5832	0.5871	0.5910	0.5948	0.5987	0.6026	0.6064	0.6103	0.6141
0.3	0.6179	0.6217	0.6255	0.6293	0.6331	0.6368	0.6406	0.6443	0.6480	0.6517
0.4	0.6554	0.6591	0.6628	0.6664	0.6700	0.6736	0.6772	0.6808	0.6844	0.6879
0.5	0.6915	0.6950	0.6985	0.7019	0.7054	0.7088	0.7123	0.7157	0.7190	0.7224
0.6	0.7257	0.7291	0.7324	0.7357	0.7389	0.7422	0.7454	0.7486	0.7517	0.7549
0.7	0.7580	0.7611	0.7642	0.7673	0.7704	0.7734	0.7764	0.7794	0.7823	0.7852
0.8	0.7881	0.7910	0.7939	0.7967	0.7995	0.8023	0.8051	0.8078	0.8106	0.8133
0.9	0.8159	0.8186	0.8212	0.8238	0.8264	0.8289	0.8315	0.8340	0.8365	0.8389
1.0	0.8413	0.8438	0.8461	0.8485	0.8508	0.8531	0.8554	0.8577	0.8599	0.8621
1.1	0.8643	0.8665	0.8686	0.8708	0.8729	0.8749	0.8770	0.8790	0.8810	0.8830
1.2	0.8849	0.8869	0.8888	0.8907	0.8925	0.8944	0.8962	0.8980	0.8997	0.9015
1.3	0.9032	0.9049	0.9066	0.9082	0.9099	0.9115	0.9131	0.9147	0.9162	0.9177
1.4	0.9192	0.9207	0.9222	0.9236	0.9251	0.9265	0.9279	0.9292	0.9306	0.9319
1.5	0.9332	0.9345	0.9357	0.9370	0.9382	0.9394	0.9406	0.9418	0.9429	0.9441
1.6	0.9452	0.9463	0.9474	0.9484	0.9495	0.9505	0.9515	0.9525	0.9535	0.9545
1.7	0.9554	0.9564	0.9573	0.9582	0.9591	0.9599	0.9608	0.9616	0.9625	0.9633
1.8	0.9641	0.9649	0.9656	0.9664	0.9671	0.9678	0.9686	0.9693	0.9699	0.9706
1.9	0.9713	0.9719	0.9726	0.9732	0.9738	0.9744	0.9750	0.9756	0.9761	0.9767
2.0	0.9772	0.9778	0.9783	0.9788	0.9793	0.9798	0.9803	0.9808	0.9812	0.9817
2.1	0.9821	0.9826	0.9830	0.9834	0.9838	0.9842	0.9846	0.9850	0.9854	0.9857
2.2	0.9861	0.9864	0.9868	0.9871	0.9875	0.9878	0.9881	0.9884	0.9887	0.9890
2.3	0.9893	0.9896	0.9898	0.9901	0.9904	0.9906	0.9909	0.9911	0.9913	0.9916
2.4	0.9918	0.9920	0.9922	0.9925	0.9927	0.9929	0.9931	0.9932	0.9934	0.9936
2.5	0.9938	0.9940	0.9941	0.9943	0.9945	0.9946	0.9948	0.9949	0.9951	0.9952
2.6	0.9953	0.9955	0.9956	0.9957	0.9959	0.9960	0.9961	0.9962	0.9963	0.9964
2.7	0.9965	0.9966	0.9967	0.9968	0.9969	0.9970	0.9971	0.9972	0.9973	0.9974
2.8	0.9974	0.9975	0.9976	0.9977	0.9977	0.9978	0.9979	0.9979	0.9980	0.9981
2.9	0.9981	0.9982	0.9982	0.9983	0.9984	0.9984	0.9985	0.9985	0.9986	0.9986

Appendix C
Percentage points
of *t*-distributions

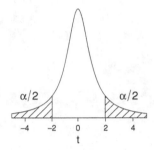

Probability $\alpha/2$ in each tail.

Degrees of freedom	α		Degrees of freedom	α	
	5%	1%		5%	1%
1	12.706	63.657	16	2.120	2.921
2	4.303	9.925	17	2.110	2.898
3	3.182	5.841	18	2.101	2.878
4	2.776	4.604	19	2.093	2.861
5	2.571	4.032	20	2.086	2.845
6	2.447	3.707	21	2.080	2.831
7	2.365	3.499	22	2.074	2.819
8	2.306	3.355	23	2.069	2.807
9	2.262	3.250	24	2.064	2.797
10	2.228	3.169	25	2.060	2.787
11	2.201	3.106	30	2.042	2.750
12	2.179	3.055	40	2.021	2.704
13	2.160	3.012	50	2.009	2.678
14	2.145	2.977	∞	1.960	2.576
15	2.131	2.947			

Appendix D
Percentage points of χ^2-distributions

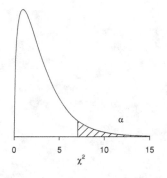

Probability α in tail, values of χ^2 in table. So for 3 df $\alpha = 0.05$ occurs at $\chi^2 = 7.185$

Degrees of freedom	α 5%	1%	Degrees of freedom	α 5%	1%
1	3.84	6.63	15	25.00	30.58
2	5.99	9.21	16	26.30	32.00
3	7.81	11.34	17	27.59	33.41
4	9.49	13.28	18	28.87	34.81
5	11.07	15.09	19	30.14	36.19
6	12.59	16.81	20	31.41	37.57
7	14.07	18.48	21	32.67	38.93
8	15.51	20.09	22	33.92	40.29
9	16.92	21.67	23	35.17	41.64
10	18.31	23.21	24	36.42	42.98
11	19.68	24.72	25	37.65	44.31
12	21.03	26.22	30	43.77	50.89
13	22.36	27.69	40	55.76	63.69
14	23.68	29.14	50	67.50	76.15

Appendix E
Percentage points of beta-beta distributions

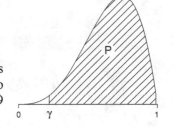

Lower limit of probability P occurs at γ for given positives and negatives and prior parameters $\alpha = 1$, and $\beta = 1$. So for 1 negative and 3 positives the lower bound for $P = 0.99$ is at $\gamma = 0.22$.

Positives	0 negatives			1 negative			2 negatives		
	90%	95%	99%	90%	95%	99%	90%	95%	99%
1	0.31	0.22	0.10	0.20	0.14	0.06	0.14	0.10	0.04
2	0.46	0.37	0.21	0.32	0.25	0.14	0.25	0.19	0.11
3	0.56	0.47	0.31	0.42	0.34	0.22	0.33	0.27	0.17
4	0.63	0.55	0.40	0.49	0.42	0.29	0.40	0.34	0.24
5	0.68	0.60	0.46	0.55	0.48	0.36	0.46	0.40	0.29
6	0.72	0.65	0.52	0.59	0.53	0.41	0.51	0.45	0.34
7	0.75	0.68	0.56	0.63	0.57	0.46	0.55	0.49	0.39
8	0.77	0.71	0.60	0.66	0.61	0.50	0.58	0.53	0.43
9	0.79	0.74	0.63	0.69	0.64	0.53	0.61	0.56	0.46
10	0.81	0.76	0.65	0.71	0.66	0.56	0.64	0.59	0.49
11	0.82	0.78	0.68	0.73	0.68	0.59	0.66	0.61	0.52
12	0.83	0.79	0.70	0.75	0.70	0.61	0.68	0.64	0.55
13	0.84	0.80	0.72	0.76	0.72	0.63	0.70	0.66	0.57
14	0.85	0.81	0.73	0.78	0.74	0.65	0.72	0.67	0.59
15	0.86	0.83	0.75	0.79	0.75	0.67	0.73	0.69	0.61

Appendix F
Percentage points
of F-distributions

Probability α in tail, values of F in table.
 All tabulated values are for DF1 = 1.
So for (1, 20) degrees of freedom $\alpha = 0.05$ occurs at
F = 4.35.

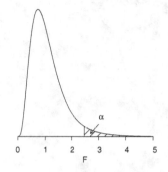

Degrees of freedom 2	α		Degrees of freedom 2	α	
	5%	1%		5%	1%
2	18.51	98.50	16	4.49	8.53
3	10.13	34.12	17	4.45	8.40
4	7.71	21.20	18	4.41	8.29
5	6.61	16.26	19	4.38	8.18
6	5.99	13.75	20	4.35	8.10
7	5.59	12.25	21	4.32	8.02
8	5.32	11.26	22	4.30	7.95
9	5.12	10.56	23	4.28	7.88
10	4.96	10.04	24	4.26	7.82
11	4.84	9.65	25	4.24	7.77
12	4.75	9.33	26	4.23	7.72
13	4.67	9.07	30	4.17	7.56
14	4.60	8.86	40	4.08	7.31
15	4.54	8.68	50	4.03	7.17

Appendix G
Calculating partial correlations using Excel software

Calculating partial correlation coefficients where more than a single variable is controlled for requires a more advanced technique than the simple Equation 14 on p. 67. More specifically, it necessitates a mathematical technique called 'inversion' upon the full correlation matrix. Inverting a matrix is a method from a field of mathematics called matrix algebra, and is an analogous operation to finding the reciprocal of a single number in day-to-day mathematics. For matrices with more than two rows and columns a computer is necessary to evaluate the inverse of a matrix. It can be calculated by hand, but can be very tricky and tedious. Luckily inversions can be performed with the commonly available Excel spreadsheet, or with many other software packages. From the example for morphine and its metabolites in Section 6.5 the full correlation matrix is:

1.000	0.818	0.920	0.399	0.163	0.206
0.818	1.000	0.712	0.325	0.159	0.174
0.920	0.712	1.000	0.379	0.105	0.224
0.399	0.325	0.379	1.000	0.009	0.219
0.163	0.159	0.105	0.009	1.000	0.538
0.206	0.174	0.224	0.219	0.538	1.000

In the correlation matrix above the variable names have been left out for clarity, but the rows and columns are the same as Table 6.9 on p. 69.

To invert this matrix first enter it into an Excel spreadsheet in the form above, that is, in rows and columns. Then select a different range of cells of the same dimensions as the matrix to be inverted. For example, if the above matrix has its top left-hand corner at cell $A1$ and bottom right corner at cell $F6$, then one might select the range from cell $A8$ to $F14$. Any range can be selected provided it has the same dimensions as the matrix to be inverted, in this case 6×6, and does not overlap with the matrix.

Then press the $=$ key; this tells *excel* that the contents of the cells are going to be a function. The function is going to be inversion which is invoked by *minverse*, so key in: = `minverse(`. The opening parenthesis suggests to Excel that a range of cells is required, so the mouse can now be used to select the original correlation matrix, or the range of cells can be typed in manually. The contents of the cell, and of the function taskbar should now (using the example above) look like: = `minverse(A1:F6`. The closing parenthesis can now be added, do not press enter/return yet.

The function editing bar should contain =`minverse(A1:F6)`. Now comes the trick. The function needs to be what is termed in Excel an array function, that is, applied to an array. To make the *minverse* command above into an array function press `ctrl`, `shift` and `enter/return` simultaneously. This should result in the range of cells initially selected containing the values:

10.484	−3.304	−7.14	−0.507	−0.699	0.502
−3.304	3.126	0.825	−0.003	−0.028	−0.033
−7.14	0.825	7.034	0.037	0.608	−0.583
−0.507	−0.003	0.037	1.253	0.230	−0.302
−0.699	−0.028	0.608	0.230	1.51	−0.85
0.502	−0.033	−0.583	−0.302	−0.850	1.556

This is the inverse of the correlation matrix. If, with this example, you have just a single cell containing the value 10.484 then a mistake has been made, and the function has not been defined as an *array* function. This is usually because the output range of cells has not been defined, or has become unselected somewhere along the line, or `enter/return` was pressed rather than `ctrl`, `shift` and `enter/return` simultaneously. The only remedy for this is to try the above instructions again from where one initially defines the range of cells which hold the output (obviously there is no need to retype the correlation matrix).

With the calculation of the inverse of the correlation matrix we are halfway there. The matrix now needs to be scaled to become a matrix of partial correlation coefficients. The scaling is done by dividing each value in the partial correlation matrix by the negative of the square root of the product of the corresponding values in the leading diagonal.

As from this point we are only interested in the upper (or lower) triangle of the matrix, the inversion of the correlation matrix, is replicated here as the upper triangle of the matrix with the leading diagonal in bold.

10.484	−3.304	−7.14	−0.507	−0.699	0.502
–	**3.126**	0.825	−0.003	−0.028	−0.033
–	–	**7.034**	0.037	0.608	−0.583
–	–	–	**1.253**	0.230	−0.302
–	–	–	–	**1.510**	−0.850
–	–	–	–	–	**1.556**

The leading diagonal of the inverse of the correlation matrix is the sequence of values highlighted in bold in the above table, and is simply the line of cells of the matrix going from top left to bottom right, and is the vector {10.484, 3.126, 7.034, 1.253, 1.510, 1.556}.

To calculate the partial correlation coefficient between the first variable and the second variable we see the value in the corresponding cell is −3.304; this is the cell in row one and column two. The values in the leading diagonal are 10.484 for row one, and 3.126 for column two (rows and columns do not really make much difference here). Their product is $10.484 \times 3.126 = 32.762$, the square root of this is 5.724, and its negative value is -5.724. Dividing -3.304 by 5.724 we have 0.577, which is the partial correlation between variable one and two *given* all the other variables.

Taking another example, for variables five and three the inverse of the correlation matrix has a value of 0.608 (row three, column five). The respective values from the leading diagonal are 7.034 and 1.510. Multiplying 7.034 and 1.510 we have 10.621. The square root of 10.621 is 3.259, and the negative of that is -3.259. Dividing 0.608 by -3.259 we have -0.187, which is the partial correlation of variables three and five given the correlations of all the others.

This scaling should be applied to every value in the table above, except those values on the leading diagonal which have to scale to -1, to obtain the upper triangle of the partial correlation table for all variable pairs, given all the other variables.

-1.000	0.577	0.832	0.140	0.175	-0.124
$-$	-1.000	-0.178	0.002	0.012	0.015
$-$	$-$	-1.000	-0.013	-0.187	0.176
$-$	$-$	$-$	-1.000	-0.168	0.216
$-$	$-$	$-$	$-$	-1.000	0.555
$-$	$-$	$-$	$-$	$-$	-1.000

The table above contains the values for the partial correlations of each variable with each other variable *given* the correlations of all the other variables. For example, -0.124 is the partial correlation between variables one and six given the correlations with all the other variables. Variable two and four have a partial correlation of 0.002 given the correlations of all the other variables (Whittaker, 1990).

Calculation of the complete correlation matrix for all variables and the scaling of the inverse of the correlation matrix is a tedious task which is subject to all manner of human errors when undertaken manually. If partial correlations are calculated frequently it may be worth setting up a spreadsheet to calculate from data entered into the spreadsheet the correlation coefficients, the inverse of the correlation matrix, and the partial correlation matrix.

Appendix H
Further algebra using the "third law"

A topic which is often confusing for forensic scientists is how statisticians derive equations for multiple joint events which consist of the product of a series of smaller conditioned statements. An example can be found on Page 165 of Evett and Weir (1998). This example is a paternity calculation, and the evidence comprises $E = \{G_C, G_M, G_{AF}\}$, where G_C is a child's genotype, G_M is a maternal genotype, and G_{AF} is an alleged father's genotype. Evett and Weir (1998) suggest that a likelihood ratio for the observation of the various genotypes given the propositions H_p and H_d is:

$$
\begin{aligned}
\text{LR} &= \frac{\Pr(E \mid H_p, I)}{\Pr(E \mid H_d, I)} \\[2mm]
&= \frac{\Pr(G_C, G_M, G_{AP} \mid H_p, I)}{\Pr(G_C, G_M, G_{AP} \mid H_d, I)}
\end{aligned}
\tag{H.1}
$$

Evett and Weir then say "From the third law of probability"

$$
\text{LR} = \frac{\Pr(G_C \mid G_M, G_{AF}, H_p, I)}{\Pr(G_C \mid G_M, G_{AF}, H_d, I)} \times \frac{\Pr(G_M, G_{AF} \mid H_p, I)}{\Pr(G_M, G_{AF} \mid H_d, I)}
\tag{H.2}
$$

The question for many unfamiliar with this sort of algebra is what use of the third law of probability turns Equation H.1 into Equation H.2?

In Section 3.1 the third law for dependent events was given as Equation 2. A more general form of Equation 2 is:

$$
\Pr(A, B \mid I) = \Pr(A \mid I)\Pr(B \mid A, I)
\tag{H.3}
$$

The I to the right of the conditioning bar simply means *any other information*. For instance in Section 3.1 we dealt with fair six sided dice. All the events referred to in Equation 2 assumed that a die was fair, and six sided, so we omitted the term to make the notation clearer. However, to be absolutely correct in our notation we should include it as in Equation H.3.

Let us now imagine the numerator of Equation H.1 as components in Equation H.3. We could write:

$$\frac{\Pr(\underbrace{G_C}_{},\underbrace{G_M, G_{AF}}_{}|\underbrace{H_p, I}_{})}{\Pr(\ A,\quad\ B\ \ |\ I\ )} \tag{H.4}$$

Using these as substitutions into Equation H.3:

$$\frac{\Pr(\underbrace{G_C}_{},\underbrace{G_M, G_{AF}}_{}|\underbrace{H_p, I}_{})}{\Pr(\ A,\quad\ B\ \ |\ I\ )} = \frac{\Pr(\underbrace{G_C}_{}|\underbrace{H_p, I}_{}) \times \Pr(\underbrace{G_M, G_{AF}}_{}|\underbrace{G_C\ H_p, I}_{})}{\Pr(\ A\ |\ I\ )\ \times \Pr(\quad B\quad |\ A,\quad I\ )}$$

The same thing can be done with the denominator in Equation H.2

$$\frac{\Pr(\underbrace{G_C}_{},\underbrace{G_M, G_{AF}}_{}|\underbrace{H_d, I}_{})}{\Pr(\ A,\quad\ B\ \ |\ I\ )} = \frac{\Pr(\underbrace{G_C}_{}|\underbrace{H_d, I}_{}) \times \Pr(\underbrace{G_M, G_{AF}}_{}|\underbrace{G_C\ H_d, I}_{})}{\Pr(\ A\ |\ I\ )\ \times \Pr(\quad B\quad |\ A,\quad I\ )}$$

Rewriting the above expression:

$$\frac{\Pr(G_C, G_M, G_{AP}\ |\ H_p, I)}{\Pr(G_C, G_M, G_{AP}\ |\ H_d, I)} = \frac{\Pr(G_C\ |\ H_p, I)}{\Pr(G_C\ |\ H_d, I)} \times \frac{\Pr(G_M, G_{AF}\ |\ G_C, H_p, I)}{\Pr(G_M, G_{AF}\ |\ G_C, H_d, I)}$$

Which is not the same result as that obtained by Evett and Weir given here in the right hand side Equation H.2. So what has happened?

Above, in Equation H.4, we selected G_C as a substitution for A, and G_M, G_{AF} as a substitution for B. We could just as well select G_M, G_{AF} as a substitution for A, and G_C as a substitution for B. So:

$$\frac{\Pr(\underbrace{G_M, G_{AF}}_{},\ \underbrace{G_C}_{}|\underbrace{H_p, I}_{})}{\Pr(\quad A,\quad\quad B\ |\ I\ )} \tag{H.5}$$

and perform exactly the same algebraic manipulation. First for the numerator:

$$\frac{\Pr(\underbrace{G_C}_{},\underbrace{G_M, G_{AF}}_{}|\underbrace{H_p, I}_{})}{\Pr(\ A,\quad\ B\ \ |\ I\ )} = \frac{\Pr(\underbrace{G_M, G_{AF}}_{}|\underbrace{H_p, I}_{}) \times \Pr(\underbrace{G_C}_{}|\underbrace{G_M, G_{AF}H_p, I}_{})}{\Pr(\quad A\quad |\ I\ )\ \times \Pr(\ B\ |\quad A,\quad\quad I\ )}$$

and then the denominator.

$$\frac{\Pr(\underbrace{G_C}_{},\underbrace{G_M, G_{AF}}_{}|\underbrace{H_d, I}_{})}{\Pr(\ A,\quad\ B\ \ |\ I\ )} = \frac{\Pr(\underbrace{G_M, G_{AF}}_{}|\underbrace{H_d, I}_{}) \times \Pr(\underbrace{G_C}_{}|\underbrace{G_M, G_{AF}H_d, I}_{})}{\Pr(\quad A\quad |\quad\quad)\ \times \Pr(\ B\ |\quad A,\quad\quad I\ )}$$

Rewriting this we get:

$$\frac{\Pr(G_C, G_M, G_{AP}\ |\ H_p, I)}{\Pr(G_C, G_M, G_{AP}\ |\ H_d, I)} = \frac{\Pr(G_M, G_{AF}\ |\ H_p, I)}{\Pr(G_M, G_{AF}\ |\ H_d, I)} \times \frac{\Pr(G_C\ |\ G_M, G_{AF}, H_p, I)}{\Pr(G_C\ |\ G_M, G_{AF}, H_d, I)}$$

$$= \frac{\Pr(G_C\ |\ G_M, G_{AF}, H_p, I)}{\Pr(G_C\ |\ G_M, G_{AF}, H_d, I)} \times \frac{\Pr(G_M, G_{AF}\ |\ H_p, I)}{\Pr(G_M, G_{AF}\ |\ H_d, I)}$$

Which is exactly the same as the expression given by Evett and Weir.

Here we have used the third law of probability to simplify a joint event with three terms to two independent conditional probabilities, one with a single event, the other with a joint event with two terms. In fact, using the substitution method above there are six different, but equal, ways in which Equation H.1 simplified. These are:

$$\frac{\Pr(G_C, G_M, G_{AP} \mid H_p, I)}{\Pr(G_C, G_M, G_{AP} \mid H_d, I)} = \frac{\Pr(G_M, G_{AF} \mid H_p, I)}{\Pr(G_M, G_{AF} \mid H_d, I)} \times \frac{\Pr(G_C \mid G_M, G_{AF}, H_p, I)}{\Pr(G_C \mid G_M, G_{AF}, H_d, I)}$$

$$= \frac{\Pr(G_C \mid H_p, I)}{\Pr(G_C \mid H_d, I)} \times \frac{\Pr(G_M, G_{AF} \mid G_C, H_p, I)}{\Pr(G_M, G_{AF} \mid G_C, H_d, I)}$$

$$= \frac{\Pr(G_C, G_M \mid H_p, I)}{\Pr(G_C, G_M \mid H_d, I)} \times \frac{\Pr(G_{AF} \mid G_C, G_M, H_p, I)}{\Pr(G_{AF} \mid G_C, G_M, H_d, I)}$$

$$= \frac{\Pr(G_{AF} \mid H_p, I)}{\Pr(G_{AF} \mid H_d, I)} \times \frac{\Pr(G_C, G_M \mid G_{AF}, H_p, I)}{\Pr(G_C, G_M \mid G_{AF}, H_d, I)}$$

$$= \frac{\Pr(G_C, G_{AF} \mid H_p, I)}{\Pr(G_C, G_{AF} \mid H_d, I)} \times \frac{\Pr(G_M \mid G_C, G_{AF}, H_p, I)}{\Pr(G_M \mid G_C, G_{AF}, H_d, I)}$$

$$= \frac{\Pr(G_M \mid H_p, I)}{\Pr(G_M \mid H_d, I)} \times \frac{\Pr(G_C, G_{AF} \mid G_M, H_p, I)}{\Pr(G_C, G_{AF} \mid G_M, H_d, I)}$$

Evett and Weir selected the first equation in the set above because they found that the first ratio of the product would evaluate to 1, thus making the evidential value equal to the second ratio.

Because a joint probability with many terms can be simplified in many different ways can sometimes lead to a certain degree of confusion as to exactly how the expression has been simplified. A way to resolve the problem is to work through every combination of terms in the joint probability until the desired expression is derived, or some useful property is observed in one of the terms.

The simplified elements can also be treated in the same way. Take for instance the last equation (above):

$$\frac{\Pr(G_C, G_M, G_{AP} \mid H_p, I)}{\Pr(G_C, G_M, G_{AP} \mid H_d, I)} = \frac{\Pr(G_M \mid H_p, I)}{\Pr(G_M \mid H_d, I)} \times \frac{\Pr(G_C, G_{AF} \mid G_M, H_p, I)}{\Pr(G_C, G_{AF} \mid G_M, H_d, I)}$$

The final ratio can be simplified:

$$\frac{\Pr(G_C, G_{AF} \mid G_M, H_p, I)}{\Pr(G_C, G_{AF} \mid G_M, H_d, I)} = \frac{\Pr(G_C \mid G_M, H_p, I)}{\Pr(G_C \mid G_M, H_d, I)} \times \frac{\Pr(G_{AF} \mid G_C, G_M, H_p, I)}{\Pr(G_{AF} \mid G_C, G_M, H_d, I)}$$

So Equation H.1 could be rewritten as the product of three ratios:

$$\frac{\Pr(G_C, G_M, G_{AP} \mid H_p, I)}{\Pr(G_C, G_M, G_{AP} \mid H_d, I)} = \frac{\Pr(G_M \mid H_p, I)}{\Pr(G_M \mid H_d, I)} \times \frac{\Pr(G_C \mid G_M, H_p, I)}{\Pr(G_C \mid G_M, H_d, I)}$$

$$\times \frac{\Pr(G_{AF} \mid G_C, G_M, H_p, I)}{\Pr(G_{AF} \mid G_C, G_M, H_d, I)}.$$

In total there are eighteen possible simplifications for any expression with three elements before the conditioning bar.

References

Aitken, C.G.G. (1999) Sampling – How big a sample? *Journal of Forensic Sciences* **44**(4): 750–760.

Aitken, C.G.G. and Lucy, D. (2002) Estimation of the quantity of drug in a consignment from measurements on a sample. *Journal of Forensic Sciences* **47**(5): 968–975.

Aitken, C.G.G. and Lucy, D. (2004) Evaluation of trace evidence in the form of multivariate data. *Applied Statistics* **53**(1): 109–122.

Aitken, C.G.G. and Taroni, K. (2004) *Statistics and the Evaluation of Evidence for Forensic Scientists.* 2nd Edn. John Wiley and Sons, Chichester.

Aitken, C.G.G., Taroni, F. and Garbolino, P. (2003) A graphical model for the evaluation of cross-transfer evidence in DNA profiles. *Theoretical Population Biology* **63**(3): 179–190.

Aitken, C.G.G., Lucy, D., Zadora, G. and Curran, J.M. (2005) Three-level multivariate data and graphical models. *Computational Statistics and Data Analysis.*

Andrasko, J. and Ståhling, S. (1999) Time since discharge of spent cartridges. *Journal of Forensic Sciences* **44**(3): 487–495.

Aykroyd, R.G., Lucy, D., Pollard, A.M and Solheim, T. (1997) Regression analysis in adult age estimation. *American Journal of Physical Anthropology* **104**(2): 259–265.

Baker, R. (2001) *Harold Shipman's Clinical Practice 1974–1998.* Her Majesties Stationary Office, Norwich.

Balding, D.J. and Donnelly, P. (1995) Inference in forensic identification. *Journal of the Royal Statistical Society: Series A Statistics in Society* **158**(1): 21–53.

Balding, D.J. and Nichols, R.A. (1997). Significant genetic correlations among Caucasians at forensic DNA loci. *Heredity* **78**(6): 583–589.

Barnett, V. (1974) *Elements of Sampling Theory.* The English Universities Press Ltd, London.

Buckleton, J.S., Walsh, K.A.J., Seber, G.A.F. and Woodfield, D.G. (1987) A stratified approach to the complication of blood group frequency surveys. *Journal of the Forensic Science Society* **27**: 103–112.

Buckleton, J.S., Walsh, S. & Harbison, S.A. (2001) The fallacy of independence testing and the use of the product rule. *Science & Justice* **41**(2): 81–84.

Çakir, A.H., Simsek, F., Acik, L. and Tasdelen, B. (2001) Distribution of HumTPOX, HumvWA, HumTHO1 alleles in a Turkish population sample. *Journal of Forensic Sciences* **46**(5): 1257–1259.

Champod, C., Evett, I. and Jackson, G. (2004) Establishing the most appropriate databases for addressing source level propositions. *Science & Justice* **44**(3): 153–164.

Cochran, W.G. (1977) *Sampling Techniques*. 3rd Edn. John Wiley & Sons, New York, USA.

Cohen, L. and Holliday, M. (1982) *Statistics for Social Scientists*. Harper & Row, London.

Collingwood, R.G. (1946) *The Idea of History*. Oxford University Press, Oxford.

Cook, R., Evett, I.W., Jackson, G., Jones, P.J. and Lambert, J.A. (1998) A hierarchy of propositions: deciding which level to address in casework. *Science & Justice* **38**(4): 231–239.

Cook, R., Evett, I.W., Jackson, G., Jones, P.J. and Lambert, J.A. (1999) Care pre-assessment and review in a two-way transfer case. *Science & Justice*; **39**(2): 103–111.

Curran, J.M., Hicks, T.N. and Buckleton, J.S. (2000) *Forensic Interpretation of Glass Evidence*. CRC Press, Boca Raton, Florida, USA.

Dawid, A.P. (2001) Comment on Stockmarr's 'likelihood ratios for evaluating DNA evidence when the suspect is found through a database search'. *Biometrics* **57**(3): 976–978.

Dawid, A.P., Mortera, J., Pascali, V.L. and Van Boxel, D. (2000) Probabilistic expert systems for forensic inference for genetic markers *Research Report 215*. Department of Statistical Sciences, University College London.

de la Grandmaison, G.L., Brion, F. and Durigon, M. (2001) Frequency of bone lesions: An inadequate criterion for gunshot wound diagnosis in skeletal. *Journal of Forensic Sciences* **46**(3): 593–595.

De Kinder, J. (2002) Ballistic fingerprinting databases. *Science & Justice* **42**(4): 197–203.

Devlin, B. (2000) Letter to the editor of Biometrics – Reply to Stockmarr 1999. *Biometrics* **56**: 1276–1277.

Devore, J. and Peck, R. (1997) *Statistics: the Exploration and Analysis of Data*. Duxbury Press.

Draper, N.R. and Smith, H. (1998) *Applied Regression Analysis*. 3rd Edn. John Wiley & Sons, New York.

Edmond, G. (1999) Science, law and narrative: helping the facts speak for themselves. *Southern Illinois University Law Journal* **23**(3): 555–582.

Eisenhart, C. (1939) The interpretation of certain regression methods and their use in biological and industrial research. *Annals of Mathematical Statistics* **10**: 162–186.

ElSohly, M.A., Ross, S.A., Mehmedic, Z., Arafat, R., Yi, B. and Banahan, B.F. (2000) Potency trends of Δ^9-THC and other cannabinoids in confiscated marijuana from 1980–1997. *Journal of Forensic Sciences* **45**(1): 24–30.

ENFSI (2003) *Guidelines on Representative Drug Sampling Institution*: European Network of Forensic Science Institutes Drugs Working Group.

Evett, I.W. (1984) A quantitive theory for interpreting transfer evidence in criminal cases. *Applied Statistics* **33**(1): 25–32.

Evett, I.W. (1987) Bayesian inference and forensic science: problems and perspectives. *The Statistician* **36**: 99–105.

Evett, I.W. (1993) Establishing the evidential value of a small quantity of material found at a crime scene. *Journal of the Forensic Science Society* **33**(2): 83–86.

Evett, I.W. (1995) Avoiding the transposed conditional. *Science & Justice* **35**(2): 127–131.

Evett, I.W. (1998) Towards a uniform framework for reporting opinions in forensic science casework. *Science & Justice* **38**(3): 198–202.

Evett, I.W. and Foreman, L.A. (2000) Letter to the editor of Biometrics – Reply to Stockmarr 1999. *Biometrics* **56**: 1274–1277.

Evett, I.W. and Weir, B.S. (1998) *Interpreting DNA Evidence: Statistical Genetics for Forensic Scientists*. Sinauer Associates Inc. Sunderland, Massachusetts, USA.

Evett, I.W., Jackson, G. and Lambert, J.A. (2000a) More on the hierarchy of propositions: exploring the distinction between explanations and propositions. *Science & Justice* **40**(1): 3–10.

Evett, I.W., Jackson, G., Lambert, J.A. and McCrossan, S. (2000b) The impact of the principles of evidence interpretation and the structure and content of statements. *Science & Justice* **40**: 233–239.

Fairley, W. and Mosteller, W.B. (1977) *Statistics and Public Policy*. Addison-Wesley, London.

Fenton, N. and Neil, M. (2000) The 'jury observation fallacy' and the use of Bayesian networks to present probabilistic legal arguements. *Mathematics Today* **36**(6): 180–187.

Fienberg, S.E. (1988) *The Evolving Role of Statistical Assessments as Evidence in the Courts*. Springer-Verlag, Berlin.

Franklin, J. (2001) *The Science of Conjecture: Evidence and Probability before Pascal*. Johns Hopkins University Press, Baltimore, USA.

Gaudette, B.D. and Keeping, E.S. (1974) An attempt at determining probabilities in human scalp hair comparison. *Journal of Forensic Sciences* **19**: 599–606.

Gerostamoulos, J. and Drummer, O.H. (2000) Postmortem redistribution of morphine and its metabolites. *Journal of Forensic Sciences* **45**(4): 843–845.

Gillard, R.D., Pollard, A.M., Sutton, P.A. and Whittaker, D.K. (1990) An improved method for age at death determination from the measurement of d-aspartic acid in dental collagen. *Archaeometry* **32**: 61–70.

Graunt, J. (1662). *Natural and Political Observations Made Upon The Bills of Mortality* London.

Grim, D.M., Siegel, J. and Allison, J. (2002) Evaluation of laser desorption mass spectrometry and UV accelerated aging of dyes on paper as tools for the evaluation of a questioned document. *Journal of Forensic Sciences* **47**(6): 1265–1273.

Gülekon, I.N. and Turgut, H.B. (2003) The external occipital protuberance: can it be used as a criterion in the determination of sex? *Journal of Forensic Sciences* **48**(3): 513–516.

Hacking, I. (1966) *The Logic of Statistical Inference*. Cambridge University Press, Cambridge.

Hodgson, D. (2002) A lawyer looks at Bayes' Theorem. *Australian Law Review* **76**: 109–118.

Izenman, A.J. (2001) Statistical and legal aspects of the forensic study of illicit drugs. *Statistical Science* **16**(1): 35–57.

Jefferys, H. (1983) *Theory of Probability*. 3rd Edn. Clarendon Press, Oxford.

Johnson, P. and Williams, R. (2004) Post-conviction DNA testing: the UK's first 'exoneration' case? *Journal: Science & Justice* **44**(2): 77–82.

Junker, K.W. (1998) Legal narratives mastering scientific narratives. *Self-image and popular narrative on science: Twentieth Century European Narratives: Tradition & Innovation*. Sixth Conference of the International Society for the Study of European Ideas (ISSEI): Haifa, Israel, 16–21 August 1998.

Katkici, Ü., Özkök, M.S. and Örsal, M. (1994) An autopsy evaluation of defence wounds in 195 homicidal deaths due to stabbing. *Journal of the Forensic Science Society* **34**(4): 237–240.

Kind, S.S. (1994) Crime investigation and criminal trial – a three chapter paradigm of evidence. *Journal of the Forensic Science Society* **34**(3): 155–164.

Koons, R.D. and Buscaglia, J. (2002) Interpretation of glass composition measurements: the effects of match criteria on discrimination capability. *Journal of Forensic Sciences* **47**(3): 505–512.

Lee, P. (2004) *Bayesian Statistics: an Introduction*. 3rd Edn. Arnold, London.

Levine, B., Moore, K.A., Titus, J.M. and Fowler, D. (2002) A comparison of carboxyhemoglobin saturation values in postmortem heart blood and peripheral blood specimens. *Journal of Forensic Sciences* **47**(6): 1388–1390.

Lindley, D.V. (1977) A problem in forensic science. *Biometrika* **64**: 207–213.

Lucy, D., Aykroyd, R.G. and Pollard, A.M. (2002) Non-parametric calibration for age estimation. *Applied Statistics* **51**(2): 183–196.

Martens, H. and Naes, T. (1989) *Multivariate Calibration* John Wiley, Chichester.

Martin, N.C., Ford, L., Pirie, A.A., Callaghan, C.L., McTurk, K., Lucy, D. and Scrimger, D.G. (Submitted). The use of phosphate buffered saline for the recovery of cells and semen from swabs. *Science & Justice*.

McNamara, J.J. and Morton, R.J. (2004) Frequency of serial sexual homicide victimization in Virginia for a ten-year period. *Journal of Forensic Sciences* **49**(3): 529–533.

Meester, R. and Sjerps, M. (2004) Why the effect of prior odds should accompany the likelihood ratio when reporting DNA evidence. *Law, Probability & Risk* **3**(1): 51–62.

Migeot, G. and De Kinder, J. (2002) Gunshot residue deposits on the gas pistons of assault rifles. *Journal of Forensic Sciences* **47**(4): 808–810.

Miller, J.C. and Miller, J.N. (1984) *Statistics for Analytical Chemistry*. Ellis Horwood Ltd, Chichester.

Montgomery, D.C. (1991) *Design and Analysis of Experiments*. 3rd Edn. John Wiley & Sons, New York, USA.

Munõz, J.I., Suárez-Peñaranda, J.M., Otero, X.L., Rodríguez-Calvo, M.S., Costas, E., Miguéns, X. and Concheiro, L. (2001) A new perspective in the estimation of postmortem interval (PMI) based on vitreous [K+]. *Journal of Forensic Sciences* **46**(2): 209–214.

Myres, R.H. (1990) *Classical and Modern Regression with Applications*. 2nd Edn. Duxbury Press, Belmont, California, USA.

National Research Council (1996) *The Evaluation of Forensic DNA Evidence*. National Academy Press, Washington DC.

O'Hagen, T. (2004) Dicing with the unknown. *Significance* **1**(3): 132–133.

Ohtani, S., Yamada, Y., Yamamoto, T., Arany, S., Gonmori, K. and Yoshioka, N. (2004) Comparison of age estimated from degree of racemization of aspartic acid, glutamic acid and alanine in the femur. *Journal of Forensic Sciences* **49**(3): 441–445.

Patel, L., Dixon, M. and David, T.J. (2003) Growth and growth charts in cystic fibrosis. *Journal of the Royal Society of Medicine* **96** (Supplement 43): 35–41.

Pittella, J.E.H. and Gusmao, S.N.S. (2003) Diffuse vascular injury in fatal road traffic accident victims: Its relationship to diffuse axonal injury. *Journal of Forensic Sciences* **48**(3): 626–630.

Popper, K.R. (1962) *Conjecture and Refutations*. Routledge & Paul Kegan, London.

Prakken, H. (2004) Analysing reasoning about evidence with formal models of argumentation. *Law, Probability & Risk* **33**(1): 33–50.

R Development Core Team (2004) *R: A language and environment for statistical computing*. R Foundation for Statistical Computing, Vienna, Austria.

Redmayne, M. (2001) *Expert Evidence and Criminal Justice*. Oxford Monographs on Criminal Law and Justice. Oxford University Press, Oxford.

Roberts, P. and Zuckerman, A. (2004) *Criminal Evidence*. Oxford University Press, Oxford.

Robertson, B. and Vignaux, G.A. (1995) *Interpreting Evidence: Evaluating Forensic Science in the Courtroom*. John Wiley & Sons, Chichester.

Rogers, N.L., Flournoy, L.E. and McCormick, W.F. (2000). The rhomboid fossa of the clavicle as a sex and age estimator. *Journal of Forensic Sciences* **45**(1): 61–67.

Scott, K.S. and Oliver, J.S. (2001) The use of vitreous humor as an alternative to whole blood for the analysis of benzodiazepines. *Journal of Forensic Sciences* **46**(3): 694–697.

Silverman, B.B. (1986) *Density Estimation for Statistics and Data Analysis*. Chapman & Hall, London.

Smith, W.H.B. (1978) *Smith's Standard Encyclopedia of Gas, Air, & Spring Guns of the World*. Arms and Armour Press, London.

Solari, A.C. and Abramovitch, K. (2002) The accuracy and precision of third molar development as an indicator of chronological. *Journal of Forensic Sciences* **47**(3): 531–535.

Solheim, T. (1989) Dental root transparency as an indication of age. *Journal of Dental Research* **97**: 189–197.

Stigler, S. (1986) *The History of Statistics*. The Belknap Press of Harvard University Press, Cambridge, Massachusetts.

Stockmarr, A. (1999) Likelihood ratios for evaluating DNA evidence when the suspect is found through a database search. *Biometrics* **55**: 671–677.

Stojanowski, C.M. and Seidemann, R.M. (1999) A reevaluation of the sex prediction accuracy of the minimum supero-inferior femoral neck diameter for modern individuals. *Journal of Forensic Sciences* **44**(6): 215–1218.

Stoney, D.A. (1991) Transfer evidence. In: Aitken, C.G.G. & Stoney, D.A. *The Use of Statistics in Forensic Science*, Ellis Horwood, London, Chapter 4, pp. 107–138.

Stoney, D.A. (1994) Relaxing the assumption of relevance and an application to one-trace and two-trace problems. *Journal of the Forensic Science Society* **34**(1): 17–21.

Thompson, R.Q., Fetterolf, D.D., Miller, M.L. and Mothershead, R.F. (1999) Aqueous recovery from cotton swabs of organic explosives residue followed by solid phase extraction, *Journal of Forensic Sciences* **44**(4): 795–804.

Thompson, W.S. and Cohle, S.D. (2004) Fifteen-year retrospective study of infant organ weights and revision of standard weight tables. *Journal of Forensic Sciences* **49**(3): 575–585.

Ülküer, M.K., Ülküer, U., Kesici, T. and Menevşe, A. (1999) Data on the PCR Turkish population based loci: LDLR, GYPA, HBGG, D7S8, and Gc. *Journal of Forensic Sciences* **44**(6): 1258–1260.

Wand, M.P. and Jones, M.C. (1995) *Kernel Smoothing*. Chapman & Hall, London.

Watkins, S.J. (2001) Conviction by mathematical error? Doctors and lawyers should get probability theory right. *British Medical Journal* **320**: 2–3.

Whittaker, J. (1990) *Graphical Models in Applied Multivariate Statistics*. Wiley, Chichester.

Wiersema, S. (2001) *Is the Bayesian Approach for You?*. European Meeting for Shoeprint/Toolmark Examiners, May 2001.

Index